Growing Old in the
Twentieth Century

This century has seen a truly revolutionary shift in the age composition of the world's industrialised countries. While fewer children have been born to each successive generation of women, more of them have survived into middle and old age and an increasing proportion of the retired now survive into their eighties and nineties and even become centenarians.

The repercussions of these changes, which are still in progress, have been varied and momentous. The magnitude of the demographic shift has generated a sense of panic in some quarters. Nightmare images have been conjured up of a society overwhelmed with the economic burden of sustaining increasing numbers of old people requiring unlimited health and welfare services and demanding unrequited servitude from their younger relatives.

Growing Old in the Twentieth Century discusses the social implications of these changes, providing an objective picture of the welfare of older people and the effect of the growth in their numbers on society. It considers the growing public consciousness of 'an old age' problem earlier in the century and the origins of present 'welfare' programmes. Also examined are dependent mother-caring daughter relationships, income differentials among pensioners, the function of old people's clubs in helping their members to maintain self-esteem, and the position of older black immigrant women in a white society.

All the essays are the result of recent independent research, most of which was sponsored by the Economic and Social Research Council and other governmental founding bodies. Collectively they provide a sober but stimulating picture for administrators, gerontologists, professional and informal carers, retired people, and all those concerned with social affairs, of the real issues which face the industrialised nations both now and in the future.

Growing Old in the Twentieth Century

Edited by Margot Jefferys

Emeritus Professor of Medical Sociology, University of London

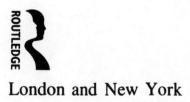

London and New York

First published in 1989
by Routledge
11 New Fetter Lane, London EC4P 4EE
29 West 35th Street, New York, NY 10001

Reprinted in 1990

First published in paperback in 1991

© 1989 Routledge

Phototypeset in 10pt Times by
Mews Photosetting, Beckenham, Kent
Printed and bound in Great Britain by
Billings & Sons Limited, Worcester

British Library Cataloguing in Publication Data

Jefferys, Margot
    Growing old in the twentieth century.
    1. Developed countries. Population Age
    structure. Socioeconomic aspects
    I. Title
    304.6′1

    ISBN 0–415–03103–6

Library of Congress Cataloging in Publication Data

Growing old in the twentieth century.

    Bibliography: p.
    Includes index.
    1. Aged–Social conditions. 2. Aged–Care.
I. Jefferys, Margot.
HQ1061.G77   1989 305.2′6   88-30665

ISBN 0–415–03103–6
    0–415–07287–5 (pbk)

Contents

Contents

Abbreviations

DHSS	Department of Health and Social Security
ESRC	Economic and Social Research Council
GHS	General Household Survey
GLAD	Greater London Association for Disabled People
GP	General practitioner
HAS	Hospital Advisory Service
IPM	Institute of Personnel Management
NCCOP	National Corporation for the Care of Old People
NCOAP (R&P)	National Conference on Old Age Pensions (Reports and Pamphlets)
NFOAPA	National Federation of Old Age Pensions Associations
NHS	National Health Service
NOPWC	National Old People's Welfare Committee
OAPA	Old Age Pensions Association
OECD	Organization for Economic Co-operation and Development
OPCS	Office of Population Censuses and Surveys
(OPCS) LS	(OPCS) Longitudinal Study
PEP	Political and Economic Planning
RNR	Relative Net Resources
SB	Supplementary Benefit(s)
TUC	Trades Union Congress
VOPSS	Voluntary Organizations Personal Social Services Group
WHO	World Health Organization

Figures

Tables

Tables

Contributors

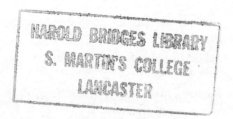
Sara Arber Lecturer in Sociology, University of Surrey.

Karl Atkin Research Associate, University of Birmingham

Frances Badger Research Officer, University of Birmingham.

Andrew Blaikie Lecturer in Social Gerontology, Birkbeck College, University of London.

Maria Brenton Lecturer in Sociology, University College, Cardiff.

Elaine Cameron Research Officer, University of Birmingham.

Angela Dale Research Fellow in Sociology, University of Surrey.

Maria Evandrou Research Officer, London School of Economics.

Helen Evers Research Officer, University of Birmingham.

Nigel Gilbert Lecturer in Sociology, University of Surrey.

Emily Grundy Lecturer in Social Gerontology, Institute of Gerontology, King's College, University of London.

Sarah Harper Lecturer in Geography, Royal Holloway and Bedford New College.

Jennifer Hockey Research Officer, Sheffield Polytechnic.

Margot Jefferys Emeritus Professor of Medical Sociology, University of London; Consultant to the ESRC on its Ageing Initiative, 1982-7.

Dorothy Jerrome Lecturer in Social Anthropology, Centre for Continuing Education, University of Sussex.

Paul Johnson Lecturer in Social History, London School of Economics.

Frank Laczko Research Officer, Centre for the Analysis of Social Policy, University of Bath.

Contributors

Jane Lewis Reader in Social Administration, London School of Economics.

John Macnicol Lecturer in Social Policy, Royal Holloway and Bedford New College.

Barbara Meredith Health and Social Services Information and Policy Officer, Age Concern, England.

Jill Russell Research Officer, University College, Cardiff.

Pat Thane Senior Lecturer in Social History, Goldsmiths' College, University of London.

Christina Victor Director, Community Medicine and Nursing Research Unit, St Mary's Hospital, London.

Alan Walker Professor of Sociological Studies, University of Sheffield.

Clare Wenger Research Fellow, Centre for Social Policy Research and Development, University College of North Wales.

Preface

In 1982, the Social Affairs Committee of the Social Science Research Council, which has since become the Economic and Social Research Council, decided that the time was ripe to take the initiative in encouraging social science research in a number of areas which it believed had been relatively neglected or under-financed. One of these areas was the wider economic, social, and cultural implications of the great demographic change in the age composition of the population which had taken place in Britain during the twentieth century. The shape of this volume of diverse papers — half of which arose directly from work financed by the ESRC — reflects that recommendation.

The introduction by myself and Pat Thane, provides a demographic overview of the major features of the changing age profile of Britain during the twentieth century and the projections for the next few decades. It considers some of the current and future implications of past changes and of those still to come, both for elderly individuals and for the wider society to which they belong. It suggests that the alarm with which the growth in the number of those aged 85 years and over is viewed reflects a deep-seated ambivalence towards older people, which can lead to an exaggeration of the size and nature of the resources required to meet their needs or of the sacrifice required by younger people. It is a matter, we argue, of our sense of values rather than of our capacity to shoulder the burden.

Part I consists of four chapters written by historians of modern social policy development. In one way or another these chapters are all concerned with either the causes and consequences of, or the financial arrangements for, the final exit of individuals from the labour force. John Macnicol and Andrew Blaikie review the circumstances in the first half of the twentieth century in which the concept of a pension to be drawn on final retirement from the work-force emerged largely to replace that of support for poverty in old age. They show how the views of contemporaries in trades unions, employers' organizations, and political parties were influenced by the then current concern with the prospects of a declining population, as well as by the depression of the national economy which marked most of the years between the two world wars.

Sarah Harper and Pat Thane carry the story on into the two decades following the Second World War. They show how ideas about old age were formed both by prevailing but conflicting concerns with the contribution which older men and women could make in the labour market, with the relationship between health and work in older people, and with the need to implement the principles embodied in the ideas of a state concerned with the welfare and financial security of its citizens from the cradle to the grave.

Paul Johnson considers the evidence used by the proponents of the idea that the economic requirements of the capitalist state in the twentieth century have resulted in a marginalization of the old and in what can be called their structured dependency. He argues that retirement from the labour force and the provision of state pensions on such retirement, rather than a method of securing the dependency on older people, has been an objective of organized labour, is welcomed by many older workers, and, with the wider availability of occupational pensions in addition to the state pension, provides older people with a considerable degree of financial freedom and hence consumer power.

Alan Walker, who is one of the proponents of the structured-dependency theory, addresses this issue only indirectly in his chapter, which reviews the fate of older workers in the three years following the closure of a large steel works in the Sheffield area in the late 1970s. He concludes that the nearer the worker was to state pension age, the more likely he or she was to take early retirement rather than seek re-employment; but he suggests that the decision was not so much a result of individual choice on the part of workers as of the virtual absence of suitable alternative employment.

The three chapters in **Part II** have two features in common: they make use of existing large data-sets and they examine various aspects of resource distribution *within* the population over retirement age. The first chapter, the work of a team from the University of Surrey, shows that the successive stages of the life course *after* retirement usually involve the transition from married status to widowhood and a cessation of earned income. Such factors, together with some cohort effects (for example, those affecting occupational pensions) rather than age itself, account for the uneven distribution of resources among households.

Christina Victor also uses General Household Survey data from the early 1980s to compare the incomes from various sources of individuals over retirement age. She argues that, contrary to a widespread belief, old age is not a leveller. Age, gender, and social class are all factors associated with income level and particularly with poverty. She traces the disparity in income levels to the life experiences of individuals.

Victor concludes that poverty among retired people, especially the very old, can only be alleviated by a more generous statutory retirement pension than the present one.

Emily Grundy uses data from the Office of Population Censuses and Surveys' longitudinal study of a 1 per cent sample of the population identified in the 1971 Census for England and Wales and followed up for registrable events such as deaths, marriages, and births occurring to 1981. She uses these data to show, for example, that socio-economic characteristics of individuals — such as their household's housing tenure and their social class — continue, for those past retirement age, to be associated with differences in survival, widowhood, and the likelihood of admission to some form of institutional living arrangement.

Each of the six chapters in **Part III** deal with some aspect of the social life of older people and/or of the relationships of those needing care with their carers. Dorothy Jerrome participated in the activities of a number of clubs, some of which were age-restricted and some open to people of all ages. The ritualized activities of old people's clubs helped to reinforce self-esteem among members, a self-esteem which the outside, everyday world threatened.

Clare Wenger, studying old people in rural communities, constructs a typology of *support* networks as distinct from wider *social* networks. The former can be dense or sparse, composed predominantly of closely related kin or of neighbours and paid helpers. With advancing age support networks are transformed, gradually or suddenly. Wenger argues that awareness of the varied structure of support networks would help social service and health personnel to make more effective plans to maintain older people in the community.

Jane Lewis and Barbara Meredith obtained information from London-based daughters who had cared for a frail or disabled mother at home to show how the caring relationship typically develops as the mother becomes more handicapped and the daughter herself ages. They emphasize the ambivalence of the emotional bonds between mothers and daughters. They believe that greater awareness of the subtleties of mother–daughter relationships would help professional carers and planners better to assess the needs of both informal carers and those cared for.

Jennifer Hockey worked as a care assistant in a local authority-run old people's home. She saw the home as a confined space in which living and dying — normally separated — go on at close quarters. Admission to the home involves acceptance of a new identity. She examined the strategies employed by residents to come to terms with their changed status, and suggests that these reflect strategies employed in the past to give meaning in their everyday lives. She attributes the broad distinctions between the ways in which men and women adjust to their changed status to the differences in the lives of the two sexes and to their experiences as exercisers or recipients of authority in public and private domains.

Jill Russell and Maria Brenton looked at the circumstances surrounding the discharge of older patients from hospital to their own homes. They draw attention to the virtual disappearance of rest homes for convalescence, which in the 1950s were often used to mediate the transition, and to the continuing failure of the National Health Service and local authority social service departments to identify and meet the needs of older people on discharge from hospital.

The final chapter, by a Birmingham-based research team, addresses what is likely to become an even more topical issue in the future — namely, the care received by disabled and frail elderly black people. They were able to interview a small but representative number of Asian and Afro-Caribbean men and women as well as white people in the Midlands who were both elderly and handicapped in some way. They conclude that the assumption that Asians are likely to be well supported by the extended family in such circumstances needs questioning. Not only does the extended family not exist at all for some older black people; for others, it is a source of tension because migration has disrupted the lives of all the generations involved.

This collection demonstrates that there is a growing body of research from the perspectives and methodologies of various social science disciplines, which is collectively, both for academic and for practical purposes, throwing light on the general and particular implications of an ageing Britain and on the quality of life of its older citizens.

Margot Jefferys
1988

Introduction: An Ageing Society and Ageing People

Margot Jefferys and Pat Thane

Introduction

In this chapter we show first how the age structure of Britain's population has changed during the twentieth century, and how it is likely to change in the century's final years and beyond. We then consider some of the current and future implications of past changes and of those still to come, both for individuals who survive into what is commonly called old age and for the wider society of which they are a part. We challenge the need for the alarm — almost panic — which the increased rate of survival of so many more people into their ninth and tenth decades appears to have evoked in some quarters. We consider the real challenges to society of having more octogenarians, nonagenerians, and centenarians in its ranks, and ask what is likely to be involved in meeting them.

The Changing Age Profile

The graph in Figure I.1 compares the age and sex structure of the population of Great Britain in 1901 — the first census of the century — with that of 1981. For 1901, the graph had the shape of a pyramid — broad at the base and tapering to the top. The pyramidical shape in that year reflected what must now be considered high mortality rates at all ages, and particularly among the very young. A comparatively small proportion of each cohort born during the nineteenth century reached old age. For 1981, the graph, representing in the main those born during the twentieth century, was more rectangular. Together, the graphs sum up what happened during the intervening eighty years. Although the birth-rate fluctuated from time to time during the century — for example, it was low in the inter-war years and high in the immediate post-Second World War years — the proportion of survivors at each age, and especially among the young, increased throughout the period. The result was that the proportion of the population over the age at which state pensions can now be drawn (65 years for men and 60 for women), increased

1

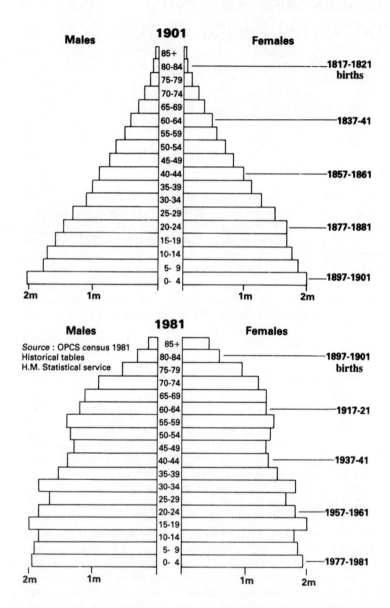

Figure I.1 Age and sex structure of the British Population, 1901 and 1981

---

over the eighty-year period from about one in twenty (5 per cent) to over one in six (about 18 per cent).

At this point it should be remembered that the proportion of the population which any particular age cohort constitutes during its lifetime is not only or indeed not mainly a function of its own initial size and subsequent mortality rate: it also depends upon the absolute size of all other cohorts and their mortality rates. Other things being equal, an increase in births decreases the proportion which all earlier cohorts constitute in the population, and a decrease in births will have the opposite effect. Moreover, the effect is perpetuated as each birth cohort advances up the age scale, especially if its mortality rate is greater or less than that of previous cohorts. This is of importance as long as those over a certain age, as well as those under another, are regarded as economically and socially dependent on the rest of the population. In Britain, it has become customary to regard those under statutory school-leaving age, as well as women over 60 years and men over 65, as dependent on the remainder of the population. The dependency ratio is then defined as the number in these age-groups as a proportion of the remaining population (Ermisch 1983) (Table I.1). Welfare economists in particular have been concerned with actual or predicted changes in the size and nature of the ratio. The dependency ratios in Table I.1 for 1961 and 1979 would be even greater if those aged 14–15 were included with the children and not with the working population. We return to this issue later.

Table I.1 Dependency ratios in Great Britain in selected years, 1901–79 (per thousand population of working age)

Year	Child[a]	Pensioner[b]	Total
1901	531	101	632
1931	365	145	510
1961	373	236	609
1979	350	284	634

Source: Ermisch, 1983
Notes: a. Persons aged 0–14.
  b. men aged 65 +, women aged 60 +

The Male–Female Balance

It is now well recognized that, in so far as survival in the twentieth century is concerned, men rather than women constitute the weaker sex. Throughout the century, rather more males than females were born, the ratio remaining relatively constant despite beliefs that the proportion of male births increases after wars in which the mortality of young adult men greatly exceeds that of young adult women.

From birth onwards, male mortality rates exceeded those of females.

Introduction

In earlier centuries, excessive child-bearing and its short- and long-term consequences took a great toll among young women, but early in the twentieth century a fall in mortality from tuberculosis, somewhat later in maternal mortality, and the diseases particular to women's reproductive functions, left males more vulnerable than females. When mortality for both sexes in infancy and childhood was great, as it was at the beginning of the century, it did not take long for a cohort to advance up the age scale before females outnumbered males. In the 1980s, it is still true that males have higher mortality *rates* than females at all ages (except possibly after reaching the age of 100 years: OPCS 1987: 5); but the *number* of deaths in childhood and early adult life is now so small that it is not until individuals reach their late forties, that women actually outnumber men of the same birth cohort. Thereafter, male mortality rates in the last decades of life have been so much greater than those for females that a significant disparity has

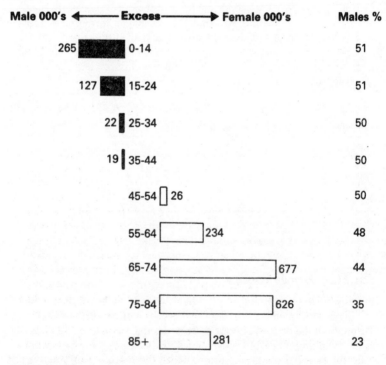

Figure I.2 Excess of female population after the age of 45 years and males as a per cent of the total (1981)

developed in the numbers of men and women in the older age-groups. Figure I.2 indicates the extent to which death continues to discriminate between men and women in older age, leaving more and more women among the survivors. Table I.2, which shows the expectation of further life in years and of *ultimate* age at various ages for men and women at various periods of the twentieth century, is another expression of their different life survival patterns and of how these have changed over time.

Table I.2 Expectation of additional years of life and ultimate age for men and women of various ages at various periods, United Kingdom

At Age	1901		1961		1981		1983	
	M	F	M	F	M	F	M	F
			Additional Years of Life[a]					
Birth	48.0	51.6	67.9	73.8	69.8	76.2	71.4	77.2
20	42.7	45.2	50.4	55.7	51.2	57.4	52.7	58.3
60	13.4	14.9	15.0	19.0	15.6	20.6	16.5	21.0
80	4.9	5.4	5.2	6.3	5.5	7.3	5.9	7.6
			Ultimate Age[a]					
Birth	48.0	51.6	67.9	73.8	69.8	76.2	71.4	77.2
20	62.7	65.2	70.4	75.7	71.2	77.4	72.7	78.3
60	73.4	74.9	75.0	79.0	75.6	80.6	76.5	81.0
80	84.9	85.4	85.2	86.3	85.5	87.3	85.9	87.6

Source: Social Trends, 1987
Note:
[a] To be expected by 50 per cent of those alive at birth or at particular ages.

Marital Status and Age

The preponderance of women in later life, especially among the over 85 year-olds (a group which is becoming known as 'the oldest old'), has also lead to another differentiating factor between the sexes in later life. Not unnaturally, there are roughly comparable numbers of *married* men and women in the population over 65 and, because men generally marry women younger than themselves, even a slight excess of males. Widows, however, greatly outnumber widowers (Figure I.3). There are also fewer never-married men than never-married women. This is partly because single status at younger ages appears to have been consistently even more lethal for men than for women. To be married is life-protective for both sexes but more so for men than for women. However, it should also be borne in mind that women, now 80 or more, belong to a generation whose chances of ever marrying were greatly reduced by the loss of eligible young men in the First World War (1914–18). In subsequent cohorts which reach the age of 80 and 90, there will be smaller proportions of never-married individuals of both sexes; the trend will be particularly noticeable for women.

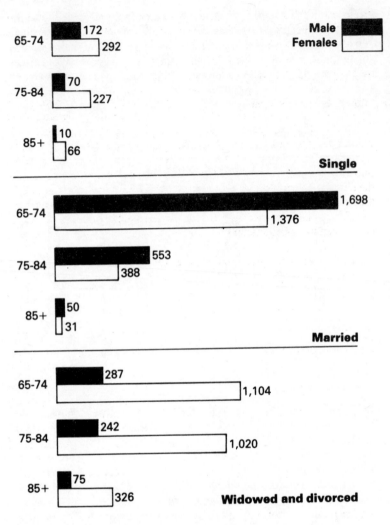

Figure I.3 Marital status by age and sex (1981)

The sex and marital status characteristics of the oldest old are important because they carry implications for personal tending if and when care
becomes essential. In the recent past and currently, the never-married,
followed by the widowed, are the most likely to require admission to
an institution in old age. The still-married are the most likely to continue
to live in their own private homes. The single too are unlikely to have

direct descendants, and personal tending is most likely to be done, after the death of a spouse, by daughters or daughters-in-law (Rossiter and Wicks 1982).

The Ageing Pensioner

One other feature of the century's demographic pattern to date needs emphasis. It is the shift which has occurred *within* the population over statutory retirement-pension age towards the oldest old. (Table I.3). Indeed, it is the implications of the changing age structure of the population *of* pensionable age and the likelihood of a continuation of that trend into at least the first decade of the twenty-first century which have been the chief concern of social planners and welfare economists, rather than the proportion of the total population entitled to draw retirement pensions. This latter has increased throughout the twentieth century; it is not an end-of-century phenomenon.

Table I.3 Number and percentage of those aged 60 and over in three age bands at various periods, United Kingdom (millions)

Year	60–74		Age band 75–84		85+		Total 60+	
	N	%	N	%	N	%	N	%
1901[1]	2.4	(83)			0.5	(17)	2.9	(100)
1931[1]	4.4	(81)			1.0	(19)	5.4	(100)
1961[2]	6.8	(76)	1.9	(21)	0.3	(3)	9.0	(100)
1971[2]	8.0	(75)	2.2	(21)	0.5	(5)	10.7	(100)
1981[2]	8.1	(71)	2.7	(24)	0.6	(5)	11.4	(100)
1985[2]	8.0	(69)	2.9	(25)	0.7	(6)	11.6	(100)
1991[3]	7.9	(66)			4.0	(34)	11.9	(100)
2001[3]	7.6	(63)			4.4	(37)	12.0	(100)
2011[3]	8.8	(66)			4.5	(34)	13.3	(100)

Source: Social Trends, 1987.
Notes: 1. Census data.
     2. Registrar-General mid-year estimates.
     3. Government Actuary projections.

The Future

There are no certainties in the field of demography, but on the assumption that present mortality rates at all ages will not worsen, we can be fairly certain about the absolute numbers of men and women over the present statutory retirement pension age (60 for women and 65 for men) well into the twenty-first century — at least until the 2040s — because all of them are already born. Unless there are radical changes in migration to and from the British Isles, or in mortality rates in middle age, or an unprecedented natural disaster, the numbers can be confidently predicted. (Table I.4).

Table I.4 Projected population of pensionable age, 1991–2051 (millions)

1991	10.4	2031	13.7
2001	10.2	2041	13.1
2011	10.9	2051	12.3
2021	12.1		

Source: Social Trends, 1987.

What is more difficult to predict into the middle of the next century is the *proportion* of the total population that this older group will constitute, because that depends upon the birth-rate, and the latter, if past experience is anything to go on, shifts unpredictably with transient social circumstances — such as the level of unemployment or whether or not there is a war — as well as with unstable social attitudes to child-bearing and the age at which it is thought suitable for women to bear children.

Although the very long-term future plays a part in present thinking (for example, concern about the burden which present promises of pension levels may impose on future generations of working age), it is the shorter-term prospects — from now until the end of the century — which mainly concern policy-makers, the caring professions, informal carers of infirm elderly people, and older people themselves. What that clearly involves (Table I.5) is first, a relatively stable total proportion over statutory retirement-pension age, but second, a substantial increase in the number and proportion of that retirement-age population which is over 85, and a decrease in the number and proportion of 65 to 74 year-olds who are now often described as 'the young elderly'. This demographic pattern was laid down in the first half of the century when the inter-war birth-rate declined markedly. Although that smaller birth cohort, which now constitutes the young elderly, had lower subsequent mortality rates at early ages than their immediate predecessors, the differences between the two have not been sufficient to eliminate the difference in their absolute numbers as they reach statutory retirement-pension age.

Table I.5 Numbers in four age bands in every thousand of the UK population in 1981 and 2001 (estimated)

Age band	1981	2001
Under 16	215	218
16–64	605	605
65–84	169	160
85+	11	17

Source: Social Trends, 1987.

The Determinants of Demographic Change

The changing age profile of Britain and other technologically advanced countries which share Britain's pattern reflects, as we have already suggested, changes over time both in the size of successive birth cohorts and in mortality rates at all ages.

The birth-rates of the twentieth century have been consistently lower in every decade than those of the nineteenth century, but there have been fluctuations. These appear to be associated in part at least with the state of the labour market and the demand for women's labour (Ermisch 1983). The sudden increase in the dissemination of information about reliable and safe contraception and abortion and their availability have also played a part in creating temporary changes in birth rates, by persuading couples to postpone rather than forgo child-bearing altogether. It is unwise to predict, therefore, either a further decline in birth-rates or stability into the unknown future.

Factors affecting mortality rates are also complex. Epidemiological research appears to favour environmental explanations for declining mortality rates in infancy and early adult life rather than medical interventions or specific pharmacological innovations for preventive and curative purposes (McKeown 1976). This appears convincing since the decline in mortality rates antedated for the most part the advent of efficacious pills and surgical procedures.

There is, however, continuing controversy about the extent to which reductions in mortality, especially in middle age and late life, have depended in the past and will depend in the future on collective measures to control the physical and social environment, or on voluntary, individualistic modifications in personal life-styles. (Townsend and Davidson 1982). The case of smoking and alcohol abuse illustrates the controversy. Both sides agree that these behaviours lead to much if not most of the premature mortality as well as chronic morbidity of adults today, and that a reduction in them would lead to reduced mortality and an enhanced quality of life. The 'structuralists' argue that the causes of such behaviours lie deep in the social organization of society, and particularly in its class divisions, and that they can only be radically modified by collective actions designed to curb the power of the purveyors of cigarettes and alcohol and to reduce social inequalities. On the other hand, the 'behaviourists' (for want of a better term) argue that the responsiblity lies fairly and squarely with individuals who are now fully informed of the dangers they face in perpetuating life-threatening behaviours.

Whatever side is taken in this ongoing debate, however, it appears that knowledge of the ill effects of tobacco has already led to a modification in smoking behaviour among older men, particularly those in non-manual employment. This, together with improvements in diet and exercise and also in the average man's or woman's physical environment throughout the century, may account for the decline in the death-rate which has continued to take place in recent years for those who have already reached middle age (see Table I.6). If this trend continues, we can expect greater numbers of each successive cohort to reach pensionable age and to have both a longer expectation of life and fewer chronic illnesses and disabilities when it does than than its predecessor. We return to this issue when we discuss the implications of greater numbers surviving into their eighties and nineties both for the survivors and for the society at large.

Table I.6 Death-rates per thousand population by sex and age at various periods (United Kingdom)

Year	Age							
	55–64		65–74		75–84		85+	
	M	F	M	F	M	F	M	F
1900–2	35.0	27.9	69.9	59.3	143.6	127.0	289.6	262.6
1950–2	23.2	12.9	55.2	35.5	127.6	98.4	272.0	228.8
1970	21.4	10.5	54.0	28.3	119.0	77.0	253.4	205.0
1975	19.9	10.4	50.5	26.0	115.2	73.4	237.2	188.3
1980	18.7	10.0	47.2	25.0	108.6	67.7	227.0	181.3
1985	17.5	9.9	45.0	24.7	104.8	64.8	223.4	178.4

Source: Annual Abstract of Statistics, 1987.

The Social and Economic Implications of Change in Britain's Age Profile

The increase in the number of 80 and 90 year-olds has been viewed with alarm by some members of the professional groups whose work brings them closely into touch with the oldest old — the geriatricians, general practitioners, nurses, social workers, occupational — and physiotherapists — as well as by others more indirectly involved (HAS 1982). Prospects of even greater longevity in future among the already long-lived have served to enhance concern still further. Particular worries have been expressed about the increasing numbers of very frail individuals in need of constant attention and of those suffering from Alzheimer's disease and other forms of senile dementia for which there are as yet no known cures. It is estimated with some reliability that one in five of those aged 85 and over now suffer from dementia (Norman 1987a: 2). if there are nearly a million of that age in 2001, then almost 200,000 will be afflicted by that time.

Some official statistics of service-use, as well as data from independent surveys indicating the extent of unmet need, serve to fuel the fire of alarm. Those aged 75 years and over use the whole gamut of health and personal social services more than do younger people, and both usage and need increase with age thereafter. Compared with younger age-groups, very old people have high consultation rates with general practitioners, and have many more home visits from these doctors — the most expensive form of consultation (*Social Trends 1987*). They constitute the bulk — and an increasing bulk — of the case-load of district nurses (ibid.: 131). The work of health visitors — traditionally and profitably with mothers and children — threatens to be 'undermined' by increasing requests from general practitioners for them to take part in the home care of the very old (ibid.: 131).

An increasing proportion of all hospital beds, not only those in geriatric or psychogeriatric wards and hospitals, are occupied by those well on into their seventies and eighties (DHSS 1987; 117–8). Day hospitals have sprung up to assist the process of rehabilitation after acute illness which can herald the onset of chronic disability and handicap; their patients are overwhelmingly the very old (Donaldson *et al.* 1986).

The home-help service, to all intents and purposes, is already a service for the very old (ibid.: 131), and so also is the meals-on-wheels service (ibid.). The number of residents of voluntary and private homes (and to a lesser extent of local authority homes) has increased, and the increase is almost entirely due to the numbers of very old entering such homes (ibid.: 133). There is a rising demand for sheltered accommodation for those who can no longer live an entirely independent life and desire some regular supervision rather than admission to a residential home. Local authorities, striving to fulfil the UK government's policy of community care, are facing increasing expenditure on such items as house adaptations, designed to promote continuing self-care and autonomy for the very disabled, among whom elderly people are prominent.

Providing services of all these kinds — and in this way also helping to supplement the personal tending work usually done gratuitously by relatives responding to the emotional bonds and obligations of kinship — can clearly not be accomplished without the expenditure of resources, human and material (Abrams 1978: 67). Also, the cost of services has to be borne, in the main, from central or local government coffers, because most older people cannot meet more than a fraction of the costs of the high levels of labour-intensive care they need.

It is generally agreed that, at the present time, there is insufficient provision to meet with dignity the needs of all those over the age of 75. If more adequate services are to be made available for the expected increase in the numbers needing them, those of working age will have to pay more in central or local taxes. Yet the heavy burden of taxation is held, in some quarters, to be behind the late twentieth-century failure of the British economy. The present Conservative government's proposals are to reduce, not increase, the taxes imposed on the incomes of the population of working age.

Therein lies the dilemma. It appears that it cannot be resolved satisfactorily without reducing publicly provided services or benefits to other sections of the population. It is not surprising, therefore, to find a widespread feeling that an ageing population is already a burden and threatens to be an even greater one in the future. It is a short step from such a view to 'blaming' older people themselves for the fiscal dilemma, another version of blaming the victim. Such an attitude is particularly rife in the USA where the youth cult has been and remains strong (Levin and Levin 1980). Unfortunately, the reported effect on some of the older generation is to make them regret having lived so long and apologize for their need to call on more services than do younger people (Norman 1987b).

Are the Right Conclusions Being Drawn?

If the picture painted in the preceding paragraphs is to be believed, it seems to follow that there are serious grounds for alarm. If survivors into the ninth and tenth decades of their lives are to be adequately served, it must be at the expense of younger generations. Does it therefore follow that an ageing population inevitably implies some impoverishment, if not among elderly, then among younger people?

There is little point in denying that if Britain is to enable the very old in the present as well as the future to live out their remaining years in dignity, more human and material resources will have to be devoted to their welfare. Older people need to be in hospital longer, to consult general practitioners more often and take more drugs, and to have more home-based chiropody and nursing services and more personal social services than younger people (*Social Trends* 1987). They also require regular long-term financial support in the form of pensions, which younger people do not receive unless they are chronically disabled or unemployed. Pensions represent a transfer of resources in the form of purchasing power from current taxpayers or pension-fund contributors to past contributors. The very young, of course, by reason of their educational needs and a societal commitment to encourage parenthood, are also more costly to the Exchequer than young adults, though not as costly as the very old; but there is the expectation that the former will, in turn, repay the resources invested in them, which is not present where the very old are concerned.

The question to be asked, therefore, is: can the nation afford to increase the resources it already feels obliged to expend on the very old? The answer, in our view, should be an unequivocal 'yes'. It is our values and not our limited means which prevent us from recognizing that our society possesses adequate resources for the task in hand. It is the way in which the public is presented with the facts, rather than the facts themselves, which almost guarantees panic and resistance to the proposal to look for extra resources.

In supporting our contention, we consider the way in which statistics are presented and the assumptions generally made about the health and dependency of older people as well as about their role as consumers rather than producers of goods and services.

The Use and Abuse of Statistics

Take first the matter of numbers. We are frequently reminded by the media and by professionals of various kinds of the size of the increase which is to be expected in the number of those aged over 75 or 85 years by the end of the century. It is less frequently pointed out that the proportion of the population of pensionable age during the same period will not increase, and that the heaviest financial cost arises from pensions, not from use of services.

Furthermore, we are usually left to infer, wrongly, that there are already fewer men and women of working age available to support a far greater number of dependents than was the case in the recent past and that the immediate future is likely to bring a worsening dependency ratio. Nor are we told that, in 1981, only eleven individuals in every thousand of the population were aged 85 or more, and that in the year 2001, their number will have only increased to seventeen per thousand. If it were put to us in this way we might be less prone to think of it as imposing a vastly increased burden on the community. Is it really so difficult for a technologically innovative and ingenious society such as ours to support seventeen in every thousand, even if all seventeen were to be in need of continuous personal care (as clearly they will not be)?

Employment Levels Above and Below Pensionable Age and the Productivity of Labour

As we have already indicated, it is generally assumed that in future there is likely to be a further reduction in the proportion of people of pensionable age who will be earning currently and hence adding to the gross national product as the latter is now calculated. At the beginning of the century, substantial numbers of the elderly population, especially men, continued to work, partly, no doubt, because they had no entitlement to a pension as of right and wished to avoid the fate of most survivors — an ignominious end in the dreaded parish workhouse (Parker 1982: 177). In more recent years, 60 years of age for women and 65 for men have tended to be the maximum ages at which permanent retirement from the labour force takes place, earnings from current employment cease, and statutory and, in some cases, occupational pensions are drawn. In each decade of the twentieth century, fewer men over 65 have been entered in the censuses as in gainful employment. Furthermore, as a result of high levels of unemployment in the 1970s and 1980s (and possibly also as a result of the capacity of the more affluent to accumulate enough resources to enable them to retire early if they wish), the percentage of those in their late fifties and early sixties who regard themselves as permanently retired has increased (Walker 1980; GHS 1986: 73; Johnson 1989).

The tendency to leave paid employment at or even before the age of eligibility for state pension may or may not continue into the future. Much depends upon the general level of employment. When it is high, employers and government welcome the labour of older workers; when it is low, there is pressure from all sides for older workers to retire (Phillipson 1982; 167). When, in the mid-1980s, over three million of those between 16 and 65 were unemployed, there was certainly pressure for those in their late fifties and early sixties to leave the labour force and little encouragement for those over 65 to stay on. It should be noted, however, that if one million of the three million were back at work and not receiving unemployment and/or supplementary benefits from the Exchequer, it would put less strain on the public purse and make it easier to meet the social security benefits for the expected one million over-85-year-olds.

Whether or not early retirement and high unemployment continue, however, they should not blind us to the need to consider other factors which influence our capacity to care for dependent populations. Thus, for instance, the productivity of every hour of work — that is, the volume of goods and services that can be produced in one hour — has immeasurably increased during the present century. One calculation, for example, showed that while the occupied population increased by 35 per cent between 1911 and 1966, the real value (at constant factor price) of the national income increased by over 150 per cent (Bacon *et al.* 1972; 64, 97). In future, given the microchip and other technological advances already in the pipeline, the trend will continue. Far fewer work-hours will be required to produce goods and services to the level needed to meet all the basic requirements for food, shelter, leisure, and health of the entire population, including the very old. An increase from eleven to seventeen in the number of the latter should not throw us! Only as long as old age is presented as an intolerable burden falling on the shoulders of the young are we persuaded to be pessimistic about the future.

The Old as Producers as well as Consumers

There is another assumption often made which needs challenging. It is that those who are not currently working for money make no contribution to the nation's gross national product — that they are consumers only, not producers. For this reason, most of those over statutory retirement-pension age are regarded as non-producers — as drones. This too, however, must be seen as a presentation of the lives of human beings, which is useful perhaps for taxation purposes but bears little resemblance to the real world. In this country, and indeed throughout the world, most of the productive tasks associated with sustaining day-to-day life and happiness — namely, child-rearing, care of the sick, and household management — are undertaken outside the field of paid employment and hence of the formal economy (Stacey 1981).

Such functions are basic to the sustenance of human life and societal cohesion. Most of them are performed by women, and most women continue to perform them into their old age, whether or not they have formerly had paid employment. If the performance were costed, the assumption that the retirement pension is not earned but an unreciprocated gift from the employed to the non-employed would be found to be untenable. In short, the older generation not only has given by its paid and unpaid labour in the past; it continues to give as well as take in the present.

In addition, it is the young old — those in their sixties and seventies — who play a major part, disproportionate to their numbers, in the maintenance of voluntary organizations which contribute not only to the welfare of the disadvantaged but also to the cultural activities of the country at large. These are by no means self-centred pursuits; they benefit society generally.

Family and Kin

Many of those whose professional work involves care for old people are prone to believe that there was once an extended family system in this country whereby successive generations of kin lived together, the younger ones caring lovingly for the oldest. They point to the increasing numbers of very old people who live on their own, and draw the invalid conclusion that kinship ties have weakened, and that obligations are no longer recognized, so that old people are left to be cared for predominantly by strangers.

The work of Laslett (1972) and others has shown effectively that the multi-generational household and an ubiquitous golden old age in the pre-industrial past are largely myths. Nevertheless, they remain strongly entrenched in both lay and professional minds. Similarly, research from the 1940s onwards (Sheldon 1948; Shanas *et al.* 1968; Wenger 1984; Wright 1986) has demonstrated that the great majority of dependent people are in touch with their offspring and receive services from them. Indeed, kinship could well be said to involve greater obligations to the old than it once did, because survivors now live longer and have fewer descendants who can share their care. Research has also suggested that older people prefer not to share accommodation with their offspring in joint households if they can no longer manage on their own. Most choose to go to residential homes rather than to those of their children.

The Survival of the Unfit

Another 'prediction' frequently made is that there will be an increase in the extent of disability among the survivors into extreme old age. It is beyond dispute that advances in medicine and improvements in living conditions have enabled individuals who at previous times would not have survived severe illness or chronic handicaps to live on, perhaps with some disability, into their seventh, eighth, and ninth decades. However, those who see the longevity of disabled people as a threat also ignore other contemporary changes which will affect the future pattern of health among the elderly (*Social Trends* 1987: 136). Medical advances have not only enabled some very disabled people to survive into old age; they have also reduced the dependency on others of very many elderly people. Hip replacements and coronary bypasses are the most spectacular examples of such advances; they increase mobility and enhance the quality of life. So can the spread of knowledge about the behaviour patterns associated with fitness in old age which has resulted from epidemiological research. There is also already evidence that healthier lifestyles at early ages — including, in particular, abstention from smoking, a reduction in alcohol consumption, more controlled eating, and regular exercise — are now being adopted, and it is probable that they will improve health at a later stage for the cohorts which adopt them. The cohorts now past retirement age, it must be remembered, had the experience of childhood during the inter-war depression years and then young adulthood in the war, when they were encouraged rather than discouraged from smoking. The legacy of those eras, which fortunately have not been repeated since, will be with them today.

We know, moreover, that the more affluent among the old in Britain are more likely to feel that they enjoy good health and less likely to suffer from conditions which restrict their mobility and capacity to participate in a wide range of social and cultural activities than the least well-off (GHS 1986; 126). There is encouraging evidence to suggest that the 'young old' today are generally both more affluent and in better physical and mental shape than were their counterparts a generation ago at the same age (ibid: 141). It is probable, therefore, that, as they age and become, in their turn, the 'older' and the 'oldest old', their health will be better than that experienced by the present generation of over 80 year-olds.

Another reason for some optimism is the increase in personal possessions with which people enter the third age. At one time it was only an affluent few who owned their own houses or capital assets which they could invest to increase their incomes. The proportion who are owner-occupiers has grown substantially, and most of them have paid off their mortgages (*Social Trends 1987*: 140). Of course, this does not mean that accommodation problems for the old are solved for all time. Other statistics, for example, show that households with retired heads have fewer domestic amenities of most kinds than younger households (GHS 1986: 67); and there is a serious shortage of sheltered housing at prices which older people can afford (Tinker 1984: 86–8). However, progress on all these scores is being made, and, if it is maintained into the 1990s, should help the oldest individuals to maintain their independence — and their health — for longer periods of time.

The Challenges

In short, statistics relating to old people are presented in such a way as to spread a great deal of gloom about the future, not only for the old themselves but for society at large. If we examine these statistics critically and the social and economic context in which changes in the age structure of Britain are likely to occur in the future, we can dispel much of that gloom. Policies and actions should not be dictated by widely held but largely unexamined preconceptions, since the distorted images which they can produce are to the detriment of ordinary people as they age.

Such a statement must not, of course, be taken to imply that the future for older people is assured if things are allowed to take their course. Those who depend entirely for their income on the state pension and means-tested income support benefits are likely to be on the fringes of unacceptable poverty unless the level of benefits is increased. Moreover, we have to make sure that older people have increased opportunities for personal fulfilment after their retirement from employment which may have been both meaningful and given them their self-esteem. In order to do this, we need to challenge many popular perceptions of old age and ageing and of their impact upon society as a whole. We need also to identify opportunities for enrichment in older age, promote them, and defend them if they are misguidedly attacked. We should remain concerned, too, with the welfare of that substantial minority of older people for whom (and for whose families) ageing has brought little joy.

One of the greatest challenges is to convince ourselves and others that the lenses of the spectacles we are usually sold may seriously distort the picture we see. The public generally should be equipped with spectacles which give it a clearer and more rounded view of the opportunities for all of an ageing Britain.

References

Abrams, P. (1978) in J. Barnes and N. Connelly (eds) *Social Care Research*, London: Bedford Square Press (quoted in Tinker 1984).

Annual Abstract of Statistics, 1987 Central Statistical Office, London: HMSO.

Bacon, R. Bain, G.S. and Pimlott, J. (1972) in A.H. Halsey (ed.) *Trends in British Society since 1900*, London: Macmillan.

DHSS (1987) *Health and Personal Social Services Statistics for England, 1987*, London: HMSO.

Donaldson, C., Wright, K. and Maynard, A. (1986) 'Determining value for money in day hospital care of the elderly', *Age and Ageing 15*: 1–7.

Ermisch, J. (1983) *The Political Economy of Demographic Change*, London: Heinemann.

GHS (1986) *General Household Survey, 1984*, London: HMSO.

HAS (1982) *The Rising Tide. Developing Services for Mental Illness and Old Age*, National Health Service, Hospital Advisory Service, HMSO.

Johnson, P. (1989) 'The structured dependency of the elderly: a critical note', Chapter 3, this volume.

Laslett, P. (1972) *The World We have lost*, 2nd edition, London: Methuen.

Levin, J. and Levin, W.C. (1980) *Ageism: Prejudice and Discrimination Against the Elderly*, Belmont, California: Wadsworth Publishing Co.

McKeown, T.(1976) *The Role of Medicine. Dream, Mirage or Nemesis?* London; Nuffield Provincial Hospitals Trust.

Norman, A. (1987a) *Severe Dementia: The Provision of Long-stay Care*, London: Centre for Policy on Ageing.

Norman, A. (1987b) *Aspects of Ageism: A Discussion Paper*, London: Centre for Policy on Ageing.

OPCS (1987) *Mortality Statistics for England & Wales, No. 17*, Government Statistical Service, London: HMSO.

Parker, S. (1982) *Work and Retirement*, London: Allen & Unwin.

Phillipson, C. (1982) *Capitalism and the Construction of Old Age*, London: Macmillan.

Rossiter, C. and Wicks, M. (1982) *Crisis or Challenge? Family Care, Elderly People and Social Policy*, London: Study Commission on the Family.

Shanas, E. Fries, H. and Townsend, P. (1968) *Old People in Three Industrial Societies*, London: Routledge & Kegan Paul.

Sheldon, J.H. (1948) *The Social Medicine of Old Age*, London: Oxford University Press.

Social Trends, 1987, No. 17, Central Statistical Office, London: HMSO.

Stacey, M. (1981) 'The division of labour revisited or overcoming the two Adams', in P. Abrams, R. Deem, J. Finch, and P. Rock (eds) *Practice and Progress: British Sociology 1950–1980*, London: Allen & Unwin.

Tinker, A. (1984) *The Elderly in Modern Society*, 2nd edition, London: Longman.

Townsend, P. and Davidson, N. (1982) *Inequalities in Health. The Black Report*, London: Penguin Books.

Walker, A. (1980) 'The social creation of poverty and dependency in old age', *Journal of Social Policy 9 (1)*: 49–75.

Wenger, C. (1984) *The Supportive Network*, London: George Allen & Unwin.

Wright, F.D. (1986) *Left to Care Alone*, Aldershot: Gower.

Part I

Retirement and Structured Dependency

Chapter one

The Politics of Retirement, 1908-1948

John Macnicol and Andrew Blaikie

In the years immediately after the Second World War, the particular concerns of old age became a subject for serious social investigation for the first time. As Sara Harper and Pat Thane indicate in Chapter 2, much significant social and medical investigation was conducted between 1945 and 1965. The growth in academic social gerontology has, however, been a much more recent phenomenon and it is only with this development that several important historical issues relating to old age in the present century have established themselves on the agenda for research. Among these we may cite debates over population ageing, the funding of pensions and other social services, and differential experiences by cohort, class, and gender. Retirement has been central to all of these, although the complexity of its impact has yet to be fully explored. Its growth is considered here as a specific political issue which, for the purposes of both clarity and brevity, is distinguished apart from the broader social history of the period.

The first half of the twentieth century saw a considerable broadening in the provision of income-maintenance facilities for elderly people in Britain such that, dragged along behind the overall rise in living standards, their absolute material conditions improved greatly. Yet at the same time, social policy and public attitudes combined to define the elderly as an increasingly useless group in society. Age-related classifications became more common; older people were inexorably shaken out of the labour market and portrayed as an unproductive 'burden' on the rest of society; and most important of all, the concept of mandatory retirement was institutionalized in the 1946 National Insurance Act. Such marginalization of older people was accompanied by increasing material prosperity and political activism. This chapter sets out to explore some aspects of this paradox. It will show that, while older people organized themselves into pressure groups and old age itself became an increasingly attractive political issue, ultimately the organizations representing pensioners found themselves powerless to combat the notion that enforced retirement should become the normal experience for older people. Their powerlessness originated partly in 'internal' factors — inadequate organizational skills, fatal reliance on labour aristocrat values, failure to mobilize a broad base of political support — but chiefly in their inability to resolve several crucial externally imposed dilemmas associated with the idea of retirement.

Retirement and the Debate on Structured Dependence

Broadly speaking, the growth of retirement in the twentieth century has been viewed in two very different ways. Radical analysts of welfare development tend to see the imposition of mandatory retirement, encouraged or enforced by state pension schemes, as part of the process whereby, in late industrial societies with highly specialized divisions of labour, elderly people are marginalized into a condition of 'structured dependence'. Peter Townsend argues that the dependence of the elderly is 'structured' in that it bears a structural relationship to social class inequalities, the division of labour, social security policies, social institutions, and so on. Furthermore, social class differences in the distribution of income and resources prior to retirement will dictate the quality of retirement as a personal experience.[1] Some, such as Alan Walker, have gone so far as to argue that 'retirement is largely a twentieth century phenomenon', and that 'the increasing dependency of elderly people in Britain has been socially engineered in order to facilitate the removal of older workers from the labour force'.[2] Others, still disinclined to imply a 'golden age of sensescence' thesis, nonetheless view the particular relationship of retirement patterns to the production process in the twentieth century as novel. Chris Phillipson, for example, recognizing the precedents to be found in earlier centuries, and acknowledging the 'historical consistency' of attitudes to older people as a reserve army of labour, maintains, nevertheless, that 'what is peculiar to our period is the scale of marginalization and the increase in the number of people directly involved'.[3]

Proponents of this view contend that it is the *intensity* of social deprivation and its institutionalization in centralized state policies, production processes, and social attitudes that constitute a sufficiently novel form of structured dependence to render it qualitatively different from reliance by elderly people on Poor Law, charity, or family in the past. Structured dependence is associated with a particular stage in the capitalist mode of production, and imposed by a paternalistic state through universalist social security provision that both protects older people and keeps them in poverty. Thus, Walker points out that, in 1981, 66.8 per cent of all pensioners lived at or below the 140 per cent supplementary-benefit level, compared with one-fifth of the non-elderly; and the risk of experiencing poverty is three times greater for those over retirement age than it is for those below it.[4]

By contrast, Richard Smith and David Thomson have argued, on the basis of long-term demographic evidence, that forms of retirement have existed throughout history and (particularly if one excludes the high birth-rate nineteenth century) that there have been many periods in which a simple dependency ratio of the elderly to the non-elderly population has been high. Smith denies that a significantly new 'problem' of poverty among the elderly emerged in the late nineteenth and early twentieth centuries. Instead, he argues, one must recognize 'a long series of endeavours to resolve persistent questions concerning the duties of the individual, the family and the community in provision for the less fortunate',[5] of which the twentieth-century saga of state pensions is but one chapter. Indeed, Thomson suggests that, in relative terms, today's pensions are lower in value than support for the elderly through the mid-nineteenth century Poor Law.[6] In his view, the advocacy of family-oriented solutions in the treatment of old age was related to phases in which 'the welfare claims on the communal funds were very pressing . . . during the periods of demographically induced difficulties'. By contrast, from 1908 to 1948 'there was a return of the collectivity to the major role in the support of the elderly . . . a swing back to a larger public than private responsibility'.[7] In other words, if retirement, in either informal or structured versions, has existed throughout history, its recent growth may simply be a tribute to its attractiveness. Leslie Hannah has argued that proof of this can be found in the growth of private pension schemes which, even if frequently initiated by employers for 'labour control' reasons, demonstrate that we have invented retirement because we want it.[8]

A number of analytical problems are raised by the rather stark polarization between these opposing views. The term 'dependence' needs deconstructing. Notionally, at least, reliance on welfare may provide certain vulnerable groups (such as single mothers) with a degree of economic security and strengthened independence. The Smith-Thomson critique offers no causal explanation of precisely why shifts have occurred in the balance of community and state provision. Likewise, tables of the age distribution in certain selected parishes in early-modern England tell us nothing about how structured dependence has altered qualitatively over time. Indeed, the central problem raised by these two opposed models is whether the qualitative and experiential features of late-industrial structured dependence are exclusive to the last half century. Clearly, unless these features are defined with precision, there is a danger of ending up with a tautological explanation: what is recent must also be novel because it is recent. Smith does not deny 'the crucial character of the transformed circumstances surrounding the elderly and their relationship with the community in the mid- or late-twentieth century', but provides no further elaboration.[9] Similarly, David Hackett Fischer maintains that growing old 'is an experience profoundly different today

23

from what it was two or three centuries ago', although the only explanation he can offer is one grounded in modernization theory.[10] Andrew Achenbaum lists four factors that have caused elderly people to emerge as a distinct social group this century — demographic trends, changing images of old age, group action by older people, and new directions in old age welfare policies.[11] Still, none of these can claim a historical distinctiveness exclusive to the recent past.

Again, these two models suggest an over-simplistic distinction between 'supply-side' and 'demand-led' factors. The former suggests that retirement spread through unfettered consumer desire for more leisure, that industrialization progressively excluded older workers but also created the national wealth and political will (through the establishment of mass democracy) to support them on state pension schemes, and that increasing personal prosperity led to the individual's growing ability to save through a private pension. The latter model depicts the imposition by an all-powerful, coercive capitalist state of enforced retirement on older workers who wish to continue in the labour market until, as in the nineteenth century, they are too infirm. In fact, neither of these two models is convincing on its own. Supply and demand are not easily separable; indeed, it is their very overlap that is interesting. As will be shown in this chapter, retirement was viewed ambiguously by working people who well realized that it distributes a variety of rewards and penalties, offering, for a minority, a period of welcome leisure in relative comfort, and, for the majority, a sharp drop in living standards with enforced idleness. While this chapter emphasizes the 'political economy' context in which the practice of retirement spread, it also stresses the point that its institutionalization did not go unnoticed by older people themselves. Their organizations had much to say, and the debate on pensions was affected by their marked ambivalence towards retirement as an imposed condition. Their relative ineffectiveness, however, was the product of an inability to resolve several cultural and economic dilemmas.

Politics and Pressure Groups

At a time when the problems of war and, later, unemployment were national priorities, it would be fallacious to talk of the existence of a 'poverty lobby', operating on a broad front and according equal status to all disadvantaged groups. Both before and during the inter-war depression, the claims of unemployed and poor families directly, if inadvertently, pre-empted the needs of older people. It would be just as mistaken to assume that pensions legislation was always indicative of concessionary responses to mounting pressure on behalf of the particular groups that eventually benefitted.[12] If, for example, one aim of private insurance was to deflect the work-force away from militancy whilst investing in human capital, trades union support for higher state pensions at earlier ages reflected a desire to create jobs for younger men whilst minimizing their own potential benefit payments. [13] Nevertheless, the study of pressure-group activity during our period shows that pensions policy was the outcome of a series of struggles which acted to curb, if not always significantly, the powers invested in successive governments.

Political theorists have drawn a distinction between 'representative' groups composed *of* interests and 'promotional' ones which speak *for* or on behalf of a particular client-body. Promotional groups will only be effective when they can deliver the full support of their clientele. On the other hand, groups purporting to be an authoritative mouthpiece may be disregarded because their membership covers only a fraction of, say, all old people. In recent years, for instance, Whitehall has refused to recognize both the National Federation of Old Age Pensions Associations and Age Concern as 'truly negotiating bodies'.[14] As consumers, but non-producers, retired people possess no strike sanction. Although alliances with producer groups such as the trades unions may be sought, the absence of independent industrial muscle renders them, in Bachrach and Baratz's terms, 'influential' rather then 'powerful'.[15]

Between 1908 and 1948 several groups negotiated the needs of older people, among them the National Conference on Old Age Pensions (NCOAP), the National Spinsters' Pensions Association (which played an important role in the reduction of women's pension age from 65 to 60), the National Federation of Old Age Pensions Associations (NFOAPA), and the National Old People's Welfare Committee, established by voluntary groups during the Second World War. For the purposes of the present discussion, the NCOAP and NFOAPA provide suitably contrasting examples: to the former we might attach the tag 'promotional', to the latter a 'representative' label. The following discussion locates the campaigning activities of these two groups in the context of changes in official pensions policy, and focuses on the crucial role of the trade unions in the process of policy-making.

Pensions and Thrift, 1908–25

Following a thirty-year campaign, during which the issue of poverty in old age was thoroughly discussed, the 1908 Old Age Pension Act was the first, and definitive, legislative step on the road to the imposition of a retirement condition some forty years later. The Act itself carried no such condition. It offered, as Pat Thane put it, 'a pension for the very old, the very poor and the very respectable' with a qualifying age of 70, a sliding scale income limit of £21 to £31 10s. per annum, and clauses purporting to exclude recipients of poor relief, those convicted of various offences, and aliens.[16] The immediate aim (in response to an increasingly vociferous political campaign) was to relieve poverty in old age, and, secondarily, to lower Poor Law expenditure on the elderly. The extent of the hidden need met by the Act was demonstated by the fact that 93.6 per cent of pensions granted in 1912–13 were for the full amount of 5s 0d.[17] Following the 1908 Act discussion centred on whether thrift could be encouraged in any way that would not be inherently counter-productive. Most of the private members' old age pension bills that had been submitted to Parliament prior to 1908 had contained income-limit clauses; but by the early 1920s, stimulated partly by the 1919 Ryland Adkins Committee's publicizing of the the problem, increasing concern was being voiced over whether means-testing would discourage saving for old age. Those who spoke on behalf of the elderly found themselves in a dilemma. Means-testing was repugnant, yet how else could higher pensions be legitimated?

Between 1915 and 1918, owing to wartime employment opportunities, the number of pensioners fell; but for impoverished elderly people, inflation did nothing to improve living standards. Politically, the leaders of organized labour were the most determined campaigners on the pensioners' behalf. In the House of Commons, their loudest advocate, Tom Wing, sustained by resolutions from local pensions-committees and trades councils, exposed cases where elderly people had relinquished their pensions and drawn out-relief instead.[18]

Such intervention was given its most potent fillip in July 1916 with the first National Conference on Old Age Pensions (NCOAP). A pressure group with membership composed of affiliates from the trade unions, friendly societies, Co-operative Society committees, the Free Church Council, and others, the Conference claimed at the outset to have the support of over ten million people. Initially, a token allegiance was offered by some forty-seven MPs from all parties. Soon, however, over a hundred were identified with the movement which, by 1917, had 'a very large and influential' Commons Committee under Wing's chairmanship.[19] Aside from the clear financial objective of an increase in the basic weekly rate to 7s 6d, the association was mainly concerned with the inconsistencies of the 1908 Act in so far as the means test mitigated against the 'respectable aged Britisher'. Sir Thomas Oliver, presiding at the first conference, remarked that:

> the time had come when the old age pension should be given, irrespective of social position, sex, and necessity, to every person in the UK on reaching the age of 70 . . . the fact that some men and women had received the pension while other hardworking and deserving people had not, created a prejudice . . . At present the thrifty working man could be refused the benefit of the OAP Act, while the thriftless could receive it . . . The passport to the old

age pension should not be necessity, but British parentage.[20]

In July 1916 there had been 978,112 state pensioners; by 1924 there were 916,771, over 61,000 fewer. Against this, the number of paupers aged 70 years and over rose from 54,539 to 80,404.[21] For a generation ostensibly reared on the Smilesian creed, argued the NCOAP, this must be an anathema: an expensive system of pauperism was encouraged whilst self-reliance was discouraged. In 1915 the National Conference estimated the cost of a pauper to be 14s 0d per week and that of a criminal 11s 10d net, but a state pensioner, 'a British subject, who is required under the Act, to be a respectable and provident person' was granted between 1s 0d and 5s 0d per week only. Campaigning concentrated on attacking the 'penalty on thrift', whereby superannuation payments exceeding 8s 0d weekly from unions and, especially, from friendly societies caused pensions to be cut or disentitled claimants altogether. To avoid similar disqualifications railway companies and others had 'most unwillingly' been obliged to lower occupational pensions, either at their own instigation or following requests from employees. As the Conference's actuary pointed out, few employers would gladly contemplate taxation to finance state provision, when, simultaneously, they were developing private pension schemes. These latter prevented employees benefiting from state provision and, indirectly, money spent by employers went to relieve the Treasury, rather than the workmen for whom it was intended.[22]

Thrift had to be seen as a goal, not an all-pervading reality. It meant 'self-respect . . . the poor man's sword of honour', a fine doctrine for 'the many deserving people belonging to the small shopkeeping and lower professional classes'. However, although it was considered a duty to encourage providence, saving was for many a stark impossibility. The providential principle was only workable, it was argued, if the millionaire and the pauper were granted equal eligibility via a universal pension-scheme.[23] However, the NCOAP directed the greater part of its invective at the moral issue, rather than at the prior financial one.

Giving evidence before the Select Committee on Old Age Pensions in 1919, NCOAP secretary Longstaff Dennison stated 'We take anomalies first . . . and then the reduction of age if possible, and then increased pensions.' Because of this declared order of priorities, intensive questioning concentrated on the issue of thrift. Were earnings to be treated in the same way as savings and gratuities? Could hard and fast lines be drawn between one form of income (or property) and another? He could but say that the only solution to such posers was a universal pension. 'You have the advantage of me', he said, outpointed embarrassingly often by the Committee's own calculations, which suggested, *inter alia*, that most were penalized on account of means alone.[24] Elsewhere, distinctions were made between self-denial, charity, and earnings, although, as Lesser remarked, the dilemma was really a moral one:

> it is really very difficult to stick to a principle when the form of capital can be changed about in the many forms that modern complex conditions will allow . . . the thing is to look at the spirit which initiates these particular forms of thrift on the part of people.[25]

By the early 1920s, however, the NCOAP's rhetoric on thrift had become, in a sense, a gift to the enemy: in November 1923 the Conservatives pledged that 'the encouragement of thrift and independence must be the underlying principle of all our social reforms', whilst in his election address of the following year Baldwin declared that the aim of 'all-in' insurance was 'to get rid of inquisitorial inquiries and encourage thrift'.[26] In no way was this inconsistent with the Ryland Adkins recommendations. Mainstream social administration opinion, inevitably constrained by fiscal orthodoxy, political considerations, and the wage structure, argued that the relaxations of means-testing which were introduced in 1924 had, in Wilson and Mackay's somewhat disingenuous verdict, 'extended non-contributory pensions as widely as the system permitted'.[27] The easiest way of advance was through a new contributory scheme.

The 1925 Widows', Orphans' and Old Age Contributory Pensions Act was thus the product of several impulses — desire by the advocates of 1924 'new Conservatism' (especially Neville Chamberlain) to forge a specifically Conservative brand of social reform in the new post-1918 conditions of virtual mass democracy, the mothers' pensions challenge by Labour, the 'all-in insurance' activity within Whitehall in 1923–4 (represented by the Anderson and Watson Committees), and the first glimmerings of realization that better pensions might encourage retirement and reduce the unemployment statistics.

The potential of pensions to reduce unemployment was beginning to be discussed within the labour movement, and was briefly alluded to by Chamberlain in the Commons debates on the 1925 Bill. The sum of 10s 0d per week for the new pension was, he admitted, inadequate but it had to correspond with the level of the non-contributory pension; and such an amount would encourage individuals to take out private pensions. Yet with contradictory logic he claimed that at this level a contributory pension would stimulate retirement, since older people would withdraw from full-time work and would 'eke out' their pensions by

> something which they may have saved for themselves or perhaps by doing an odd job here and there, and working a day or two a week,

which will not make too great demands on their strength, but will just keep the household going.[28]

If such complacent thinking brought popular credibility to those in power, NCOAP policy was best tactically misguided and at worst symptomatic of a stubborn refusal to encounter poverty rather than pauperism. When we consider the impact of state welfare on personal saving, the social base of the NCOAP — or National Conference of Representatives of Friendly Societies, Trade Unions, Associations, Federations and Councils, to use the full title — lends a telling undercurrent of motive. Henry Lesser, its vice-chairman, commented that 'the National Conference was really originated by thrift societies, whether Friendly Societies or any other societies that encourage thrift'.[29] Indeed, those exemplars of working-class respectability, the friendly and approved society officials, who comprised the mainstay of their membership, were suffering a crisis of confidence.

Recent econometric evidence offered by Paul Johnson suggests that state pensions actually resulted in increased working-class savings, along the lines predicted by Booth, but that a decline in working-class assets held in friendly societies occurred, specifically during the five years from 1916 to 1921. He emphasizes that this was a time when the significance of the 'economic security and social esteem hitherto associated with membership' was declining.[30] Hence, the notion of thrift carried little meaning: it was essentially part of a bourgeois economic outlook largely incompatible with proletarian living conditions.

The aged had, nevertheless, acquired 'a definite status in the community . . . and the 'pauper taint' [was] removed by a system of personal thrift orgainized by the state', a provision for which the Conference congratulated itself, claiming to have succeeded because it had placed national interests over and above political tactics.[31] Yet it is evident that the timing of the Act had been determined by Churchill's desire to popularize his first budget and, with the rate of pension remaining static despite inflation, the continuing poverty of many elderly people merely testified to the inefficacy of such posturing in a climate of financial stringency. In 1919, Longstaff Dennison had claimed that the NCOAP was going to be 'a trade union for pensioners'.[32] In 1926, on any economic criterion, they still had a long way to go, when, pacified by the placebos of the previous year, they claimed a moral victory, and vanished into the archives of oblivion. If a group claiming to speak on behalf of elderly people had failed to deliver because its own interests were at variance with those of its wider public, the absence of any promotional or representative body during the following decade rendered the pensioners' position still more hazardous.

Pensions and the Depression, 1925–39

The subsequent depression-hit fifteen years was a period of very slow progress in welfare innovation, particularly in the case of pensions. In 1935, the very same Neville Chamberlain, who ten years earlier had even been considering a contributory earnings-related scheme, could tell the Conservative Party annual conference that better retirement pensions would be prohibitively costly, would release only a paltry number of jobs and would create grave legal and administrative problems in enforcing the retirement condition: 'Are you going to create a new penal offence — the offence of doing work?' he asked.[33]

However, within the labour movement, interest in mandatory retirement was growing. Many trade unionists, acutely sensitive to wage reductions at a time of high unemployment and deflation, held two important views on the matter of pensions. The first was that payment of 10s 0d per week by the state to pensioners still at work encouraged employers to pay correspondingly lower wages to that section of the work-force. Thus, while trade unionists wished old people to be kept at a level of economic decency, they realized at the same time that pensions without a retirement condition would erode the wage structure and weaken trade union bargaining. John Wheatley had argued as much in the Second Reading of the 1925 Bill, while at the same time criticizing the sum of 10s 0d as inadequate.[34] Again, the TUC General Council made the same accusation when it met the Beveridge Committee seventeen years later: F.H. Wolstencroft said:

> We find it surprising, the number of members in the particular craft immediately they were 65 they were 2½d per hour worse workmen than they were before. They could only retain their job if they accepted a reduction of 2½d per hour. It worked out at the 10s 0d a week pension. We call that unfair.

This was also the view of the NFOAPA, who cited particular cases to Beveridge.[35]

Secondly, from the late 1920s onwards, retirement as an immediate and simple palliative to the problem of unemployment was increasingly debated within reformist circles. Evolving his own version of the Independent Labour Party's 'Socialism in Our Time' reflationary strategy, Oswald Mosley, when a member of the 1929 Labour government, proposed a new retirement pension. He eventually incorporated this idea into his wider plan for tackling unemployment, the 1930 Mosley Memorandum. Though rejected by the Labour Cabinet and the Treasury as impractical and contrary to the tenets of the prevailing fiscal orthodoxy, the notion of generous pensions with a retirement condition did appeal to moderate Labour opinion for the rest of the 1930s.[36] Ernest Bevin's 1933 articles in *The New Clarion*, later published as *My Plan for 2,000,000 Workless*, argued that a new state pension of £1 per week (single person) and £1 15s 0d per week (married couple) paid at the age of 65 to all earning up to £1,000 per annum, on condition of retirement from work, would induce withdrawal from the labour market of the estimated 350,000 existing pensioners aged 65–9 working in industry. If to this were added the effects of a special pension at 60 for those who were unemployed, a new invalidity pension, the raising of the school-leaving age to sixteen and a uniform forty-hour week, a total of 2,000,000 jobs would be redistributed to the unemployed.[37]

Bevin's plan was only one of a number of retirement pension schemes discussed in the 1930s. On 21 February 1934, for example, the House of Commons spent three and a half hours considering John Banfield's motion for state pensions at age 60 'sufficient in amount to encourage the retirement from industry' of older workers. It was rejected on grounds of cost and the problem of enforcing the retirement condition.[38]

Probably the most systematic exposition of such a proposal in the 1930s came from the research organization Political and Economic Planning (PEP). Formed in the aftermath of the 1931 financial crisis, PEP exemplified that liberal-reformist strand of 'middle opinion' that was to grow in the 1930s and provide the basis for the political shift leftwards during the Second World War. A moderate reform of capitalism could, it was argued, be effected through a rational planning programme. Hence, it was not surprising that, as an answer to the problem of unemployment, PEP should have seized upon the seductively plausible idea of retirement pensions that had originated in Labour circles ten years earlier.

Under its 1935 plan, PEP identified a total population aged 65 and over of 3,316,453. Of these, 837,905 were 'gainfully occupied' (this term included unemployed, casual, and part-time workers), of which 693,624 individuals were in work; 2,097,146 men and women aged 65 and over were in receipt of old age pensions (and about one-tenth of these also received public assistance). Compulsory retirement, PEP considered, would be a political impossibility since it would interfere with individual liberty, not to speak of raising the anomaly of those in occupations with no statutory upper age-limit, such as judges. However, a pension of 15s 0d per week at the age of 65, conditional on retirement (plus an equal amount for wives), would probably remove 316,000 individuals from employment at an annual cost of about £20,000,000.[39] Proposals such as these aroused considerable debate in the 1930s (particularly on the question of whether, for every job vacated by an older worker, a new one would be created for a younger person), but they made little headway with the National Government.

Jam Today! The Politics of the NFOAPA, 1938–48

Unlike earlier efforts, pressure-group agitation during the late 1930s and 1940s owed much to the militancy of pensioners themselves. From small beginnings the Old Age Pensions Association (OAPA) mushroomed. The Blackburn branch, founded in October 1938 with nine members, grew to 3,500 by February 1940, whilst even small branches, such as Rhymney in South Wales, had 360 adherents by this time. By mid-1940 their mouthpiece, *The Pensioner*, claimed sales in excess of 500 in several branches and reported on the 'phenomenal growth' of the movement — to 600 branches — within its first sixteenth months. Meanwhile, the Scottish OAPA, formed in February 1937, comprised a total membership of 8,000 by the start of 1941.[40] Following splits and amalgamation, the NFOAPA, as it became, comprised some 400 branches by June 1942. In August it was remarked in the Commons that, 'Wherever you go now in every constituency you are met by the aged people and their organizations.' By Spring 1944 some branches had nearly 10,000 members, and many had over 5,000. In villages like Dearham in Cumberland, with a total population of 1,500, 900 were members of the Federation.[41]

Such growth owed much to the sense of purpose and national identity gained through petitioning Parliament. The first petition, in July 1939, asked for a doubling of the basic pension to £1, and collected an estimated five million signatures during six weeks of local canvassing. The Speaker of the House of Commons remarked: 'This is a historic occasion. It is the first time in the history of this House that a petition has been presented accompanied by a demand.' This was a long way from the 'silent suffering' and 'passive protest' which the NCOAP had sought to articulate.[42]

Concessions gained during wartime followed a similarly piecemeal path to those granted after NCOAP pressure during the 1914–19 period. Like the NCOAP, the Federation was non-partisan, but, unlike its predecessor, its hands were not tied by affiliation to (and therefore responsibility for) the friendly society or trade union movement. This openness, together with the decentralized branch network, enabled initiatives to come 'from below', from the elderly themselves. Undoubtedly, there were echoes of an earlier campaigning style, but the rhetoric of the Federation — as reflected in the pages of *The Pensioner* — was altogether more direct and biting, more tangible. One issue cited a *Daily Herald* report on Nazi Germany which claimed that 'About 40,000 prisoners are between 65 and 85 years old. They live in barracks . . . and are allowed a shilling a day upkeep. *On this meagre subsistence allowance they die like flies*'. 'So what?', said the Federation, having shown by budgetary analysis that British pensioners also fared on just 7/- a week after rent and fuel costs had been paid.[43] Their immediate reaction to the Beveridge Report's proposals was displayed graphically in a cartoon, the caption to which read 'Cheer up, Maggie, we shall get £2 a week when we are 97 — a bitter comment on the gradualist compromises of the new pension scheme.[44] A Pensioners' National Appeal had been taken up by the *Daily Dispatch* in 1938 and Ritchie Calder's articles in the *Daily Herald*, 'Life on 10/- a Week', provided a further boost for the 1939 agitation with their Orwellian revelations.[45]

In keeping with the rank-and-file strength of the movement, however, pressure was applied most effectively at local level. By comparison with the 'insider' methods of the Old People's Welfare Committees, it was also profoundly political, resembling, as later commentators put it, 'the abrasive approach of 1960s pressure groups such as Shelter rather than the more staid "non political" approach' of the voluntary organizations.[46] Given the qualified sucess of the 1939 escapade, *The Pensioner* remarked in April 1940 that 'To exert pressure on the Govenment as a whole is to invite failure as is demonstrated by the fate of many petitions.' The point was regularly reiterated, passing resolutions being decried as equally counter-productive. Since 'not the Government, only persons can have responsibility', the struggle was to be waged in the constituencies, against individual MPs. 'We must carry on our guerilla warfare, sniping our members with postcards and letters', read the first editorial.[47]

Centralization of authority within the parties was seen as the major obstacle to the implementation of their demands. According to the National Federation, this was clearly evident from Labour's record over the past twenty years:

> One would think that, after all that time, a movement that really desired increased pensions and had failed, would have changed its tactics . . . the stronger a movement becomes "institutionally" the weaker it becomes as an instrument for the benefit of the people.[48]

All hinged on accountability. Branches engaged in detailed correspondence with local MPs, demanding an explanation from them, if Federation demands — £1 (later, 30s 0d) at 60 with no means test — were not being pursued. Several held public meetings where local MPs were put on their mettle and remorselessly pilloried if they failed to acquiesce. *The Pensioner* was, however, careful to note that 'it's the votes in Parliament that show up your MP, NOT WHAT HE SAYS ON THE PLATFORM.' The division on the Determination of Needs Bill debate in February 1941 was reprinted from Hansard, citing all 173 who had voted for the continuance of means calculations together with the 'sincere few' (nineteen) who had been carpeted for defying the Labour whip.[49] This was a tactic borrowed from the NCOAP.

However, the Federation used its local mass support to carry the campaign further. In 1943, the annual conference carried a motion suggesting all local branches put forward their own candidates for municipal elections. Subsequently, Ernest Melling (now the Federation's secretary) stood for Blackburn's staunchly Labour Trinity ward on a pensioner's independent ticket. In the 1945 general election, a mass meeting of 1,200 pensioners endorsed Barbara Castle and John Edwards, 'not because they are Labour candidates, but because they will support YOU'.[50] In addition, between 1943 and 1948 several huge mass petitions were delivered to Westminster whilst the National Council of the Independent Labour Party decided 'to place the whole machinery of the Party at the disposal of the old folk'. In April 1944 an executive deputation to London met Liberals, Tories, the *Daily Herald*, and the Assistance Board, all within the space of two days.[51]

In terms of consciousness-raising, their uncompromising approach surely paid dividends. However, the failure to influence policy decisions to the advantage of older people became painfully clear when the Beveridge Committee on Social Insurance and Allied Services examined the question of old age.

The Impact of Beveridge

Almost as soon as he commenced taking evidence, Beveridge was inundated with memoranda on the needs of the elderly. Thus, for example, the National Council of Social Service submitted a wide-ranging document summarizing the principal issues: the deficiencies in existing pensions coverage (such as the continued operation of means-testing through the 1940 supplementary pensions scheme), the urgent need for better medical assistance for pensioners outside the Public Assistance Committee services, the lack of institutional provision, and so on.[52]

It is clear, however, that Beveridge paid scant attention to these wider issues. His focus — no doubt justifiable by the Committee's terms of reference — was limited: to the establishment of a single pension integrated into the new social insurance scheme, and the reduction of supplementation by the Assistance Board. Also, his attitude towards old age was, to say the least, brisk and unsentimental. Though rejecting the more extreme nostrums of the eugenists, Beveridge had become very interested in the population problem and had written much on the question of declining fertility. He accepted uncritically the simplistic concept of a worsening dependency ratio that had been popularized in Enid Charles's alarmist warnings, for repeatedly he portrayed the elderly as a social burden and welcomed any suggestion that would limit the future cost of pensions. Thus, for example, when meeting the TUC General Council in January 1942 he warned that he could not put money towards the elderly 'at the cost of the children' and that he had to give them 'fair treatment without ruining the country'.[53] Again, in March 1942, he told the Parliamentary Committee of the Co-operative Congress that 'old age is going to be frightfully expensive; there are going to be a fearful lot of old people'.[54]

Given his attitude, then, Beveridge was likely to be favourable towards a retirement condition. The curious fact is, however, that initially he seems to have been opposed to it, and, in altering his position, was largely persuaded by the TUC General Council. Even more than in the 1930s, the TUC were imprisoned within constraints imposed on it by a capitalist wage-structure: the TUC argued strongly for adequate pensions (denying, for example, that an old person needed less to eat); but if this was to be implemented without encouraging further wage-cuts to elderly workers, then it appeared to them inevitable that a retirement condition must be introduced.

In his first major memorandum to the committee (the famous *Basic Problems of Social Security with Heads of a Scheme*), Beveridge argued that the crux of the problem was to raise pensions sufficiently to dispense with means-tested supplementation from the Assistance Board (so that the insurance basis for the entire social security plan would not be eroded), and concluded that 'these pensions will be paid on proof of age, without means test and without proof of disability or retirement from work'.[55] In his first meeting with the TUC General Council in January 1942, Beveridge rejected their suggestion for a retirement condition, saying 'I do not believe the old people leaving the labour market really create fresh employment', but he promised to look further into the matter.[56] By February he was at least considering a retirement condition, though still sceptical about its effect on unemployment, and commissioned a paper on the feasibility of enforcing it from the Ministry of Labour's representative on the Committee, P.Y. Blundun. By May, meeting the TUC again, he found their suggestion 'very interesting and attractive', but was apprehensive that any consequent investigation of whether the pensioner had worked in the previous week would smack of means-testing.[57] The TUC were insistent, however, that pensioners should make room for younger workers and that retirement should be a time of genuine leisure on an adequate payment from the state as a reward for a lifetime's work. Indeed, on this point they were the most vehement of the groups that gave evidence to the Beveridge Committee. The British Employers' Confederation, for example, had no strong views on the matter, the NFOAPA vaguely opposed compulsory retirement, and only the Fabian Society had given it much thought: they proposed an interesting 'double-decker' scheme, involving payment of 10s 0d per week as in the existing system, and 'adequate' pensions on retirement.

By the time Beveridge drafted the section of his Report on 'The Problem of Age' in August 1942, his ideas had been formulated. He displayed perfectly that contradiction of attitude (or 'supreme paradox', as Phillipson puts it)[58] in 'expert' thinking on old age that had emerged by the 1940s — on the one hand portraying the elderly as a disastrous burden on society (men over the age of 65 and women over 60 had formed 6.2 per cent of the British population in 1901, an estimated 12.0 per cent in 1941, and would be 20.8 per cent in 1971),[59] yet on the other hand, paying lip-service to their status as an exceptionally deserving group: 'Provision made for age must be satisfactory; otherwise great numbers may suffer. On the other hand, every shilling added to pension rates is extremely costly in total . . . it is dangerous to be in any way lavish to old age.'[60]

Subsistence pensions, at 40s 0d for a married couple or 24s 0d for a single person, were only to be attained after twenty years of slowly rising rates. Meanwhile, means-tested assistance supplementation would have to continue.[61] Subsistence pensions could only be paid on retirement; failure to do this 'would impose an unjustifiable and harmful burden on all citizens below that age'.[62] Yet paradoxically, the conditions governing award of a pension should encourage the older people to continue working in order to reduce the total cost of pensions, and thus the scheme adjusted to the differing capacities of individuals to work in old age.[63] Accordingly, postponement of retirement would be rewarded by an increased pension.

That Beveridge viewed the elderly with a notable lack of sympathy is evident in the few telling phrases which appeared in the final draft of August 1942 but were left out of the published Report: to give full subsistence pensions 'as a birthday present' to an individual attaining the age of 60 or 65 would be 'reprehensible extravagance' which was 'wholly unjustifiable'. Where, in the Report, Beveridge talked of the 'strong public opinion' in favour of subsistence pensions,[64] in the private memorandum he contemptuously dismissed this as 'sentimental and political', insisting that the state should retain the right to reduce pensions below subsistence on grounds of financial stringency or a fall in the cost of living, and warning of the dangers of a 'birthday present' mentality if there was no retirement condition.[65]

Meanwhile, as Means and Smith point out, the NFOAPA's concentration on pensions issues caused it to ignore inadequacies in medical and social provision whilst 'its campaigning style was unlikely to have been appreciated' within the corridors of power.[66] Not surprisingly, when the Report was published, the Federation's leaders were far from satisfied: 'For all practical purposes, the Beveridge Report is useless . . . and we had better ignore it entirely, concentrating on action which will secure our just rights — AND NOW — not at some vague future time.' They went on to deride the 'screaming headlines', 'spate of glorification', and 'premature eulogies' which followed in its wake. They were perhaps justified in their anger at the relatively low priority accorded to older people. Their complaint that they had been betrayed by a Committee 'set up as a result of the pressure by the NFOAPA upon individual MPs' was, however, some way wide of the mark.[67]

Conclusion

By the 1940s, retirement had been written in to state support for the elderly and, as such, became part of a new institutionalized dependence. For the first time, a receipt of a pension forced an individual to relinquish the right to work. The decline in economic activity among men aged over 65 progressed steadily throughout the century — from roughly two-thirds in the 1900s to one-third in the early 1950s and less than a fifth in the 1970s. However, it is doubtful whether state pensions policies were the prime cause of this decline since it continued at much the same rate after 1948 as it had done before. Thus, when considering the impulses behind such a transformation, both supply and demand factors should be accorded equal significance. General 'political economy' explanations must be correct in locating such developments within complex shifts in the production process, industrial infrastructure, and labour force requirements occurring at a particular stage of advanced industrialization — though much work needs to be done to define these shifts more precisely.[68] On the other hand, political demands and the desire of citizens for leisure in old age were also important, and possibly there was a causal connection with the growth of paid holidays and a shorter working week.

This necessarily brief account has concentrated on the debate over the retirement condition between 1908 and 1948, and the curious 'complicity' of the labour movement in demanding a measure that was to confirm the economic uselessness of old people. Yet it is clear that TUC leaders were trapped within constraints not of their making. If they were both to preserve a measure of control over the wage structure in a capitalist economy and to win adequate state pensions for their members, then a retirement condition was inevitable. As the twentieth-century economy became more specialized, older workers were increasingly occupying positions in industry that involved unskilled, light work, or were clinging to jobs in outmoded, labour-intensive enterprises such as agriculture. This tendency was, of course, greatly exacerbated by the mass unemployment of the inter-war years. Older workers were a highly vulnerable section of the work-force, and could offer little resistance to wage cuts. To protect its younger members the TUC had to sacrifice the economic freedom of working pensioners, while through Beveridge's rationalizing, the state retained a flexible reserve army of labour in the younger elderly.

Pressure groups for the older persons were caught in a similar dilemma. The NCOAP began by pressing a universalist demand but was eventually forced to accept a compromise which, although in line with working-class notions of respectability, did not reflect the absolute material wants of the many. A generation later, the National Federation more nearly incorporated mass demands through grass-roots support. Such new, articulate expression may have derived from the fact that older people in the late 1930s comprised the first fully literate generation and were also members of a cohort which had 'acquired trade union habits and organisation'. The contributory pension lent a unifying status, making them no longer the (passive) 'aged poor' but dignified and active 'old age pensioner'. Nonetheless, their pleas still went unanswered.[69] Meanwhile, in relying on projected trends in age structure, Beveridge forecast a certain level of dependent poverty, but failed to address the generational variations in lifetime patterns of personal economic behaviour which helped to create it.

The imposition of the retirement condition constituted a novel form of institutionalized dependence. Pensions policy accompanied long-term labour-market trends, which increasingly confirmed the economic irrelevance of elderly workers. However, this was not achieved with the total acquiesence of all older people. Their organizations, and those of the labour movement, trod the tightrope of the central dilemma contained in the notion of retirement — that old age should be, on the one hand, a period of dignified leisure, adequately financed by the state as a reward for a lifetime of work, and yet, on the other, a phase in which the freedom to participate in economic life was not denied.

Notes

1. Peter Townsend, 'The structured dependency of the elderly: a creation of social policy in the twentieth century', *Ageing and Society* 1 (1) (March 1981): 5–28.
2. Alan Walker, 'Social policy and elderly people in Great Britain: the construction of dependent social and economic status in old age', in Anne-Marie Guillemard (ed.) *Old Age and the Welfare State*, (London: Sage Publications, 1983, pp. 143–67 (pp. 52, 163); Alan Walker, 'Towards a political economy of old age', *Ageing and Society* 1 (1) (March 1981): 73–94. For an overview of equivalent developments in the United States, see William Graebner, *A History of Retirement: the Meaning and Function of an American Institution, 1885–1978*, New

Haven: Yale University Press, 1980.

3. Chris Phillipson, *Capitalism and the Construction of Old Age*, London: Macmillan, 1982, pp. 7, 38.

4. Alan Walker, 'Pensions and the production of poverty in old age', in Chris Phillipson and Alan Walker (eds), *Ageing and Social Policy. A Critical Assessment*, London: Gower, 1986, pp. 184–216 (pp. 185–6).

5. Richard M. Smith, 'The structured dependence of the elderly as a recent development: some sceptical historical thoughts', *Ageing and Society* 4(4) (December 1984): 409–28 (p. 422).

6. David Thomson, 'The decline of social welfare: falling state support for the elderly since Victorian times', *Ageing and Society* 4(4) (December 1984): 451–82.

7. Smith, op. cit., pp. 422–3.

8. Leslie Hannah, *Inventing Retirement: the Development of Occupational Pensions in Britain*, Cambridge: Cambridge University Press, 1986.

9. Smith, op. cit., p. 425.

10. David Hackett Fischer, *Growing Old in America*, New York: Oxford University Press, 1977, p. 3.

11. W. Andrew Achenbaum, *Shades of Gray: Old Age, American Values and Federal Policies since 1920*, Boston: Little, Brown and Co., 1983, pp. 14–18.

12. Paul Whiteley and Steve Winyard, 'Influencing social policy: the effectiveness of the poverty lobby', *Journal of Social Policy* 12 (1) (January 1983): 1–26.

13. Roy Hay, 'Employers and social policy in Britain: the evolution of welfare legislation, 1905–14', *Social History* 4 (January 1977): 435–55 (p. 455).

14. Whiteley and Winyard, op. cit., p. 12.

15. Peter Bachrach and Morton S. Baratz, *Power and Poverty*, Oxford: Oxford University Press, 1970, and 'The two faces of power', *American Political Science Review* 56 (1962): 947–52.

16. Pat Thane, 'Non-contributory versus insurance pensions, 1878–1908', in Pat Thane (ed.) *The Origins of British Social Policy*, London: Croom Helm, 1978, pp. 84–106 (pp. 103–4).

17. Sir Arnold Wilson and G.S. Mackay, *Old Age Pensions: an Historical and Critical Study*, London: Oxford University Press, 1941, pp. 54–5.

18. *House of Commons Debates*, 5s, Vol. 78, 25 January 1916, Col. 1054; Vol. 81, 21 March 1916, Col. 36; 18 April 1916, Col. 2210; 9 April 1916, Col. 2334; Vol. 82, 4 May 1916, Cols 120–1; 30 May 1916, Cols 2563–4, 2576; Vol. 84, 11 July 1916, Col. 277.

19. *National Conference on Old Age Pensions Reports and Pamphlets* (hereafter *NCOAP R & P*), 1 July 1916, p. 1; 24 February 1917, p. 2; 8 August 1917, p. 4. The Secretary, later giving evidence before the Departmental Committee on Old-Age Pensions *Parliamentary Papers* (hereafter *PP*) 1919, Cmd. 411, Vol. 27, Appendix, *Minutes of Evidence*, Q. 1539, p. 64), claimed that 'upwards of 300 or 400' attended each conference.

20. NCOAP R & P, 1 July 1916, pp. 1–2.

21. *NCOAP R & P*, 19 August 1916, p. 2; 18 October 1924, p. 2.

22. *NCOAP R & P*, 1 December 1923, p. 2; 3 October 1920, p. 1; 19 August 1916, p. 4; *House of Commons Debates*, 5s, Vol. 91, 8 March 1917, Cols 669–70.

23. *NCOAP R & P*, 1 December 1923, p. 4; 19 August 1916, p. 1; 23 February 1918, p. 5.

24. *PP* 1919, op. cit., Q. 1053, p. 46; Q. 1026, p. 45; Q. 1034, p. 45; Q. 1217, p. 52; Q. 1414, p. 60 and see pp. 43–61, 62–4 for Longstaff Dennison's evidence.

25. Ibid., Qs 2710–14, p. 108; Qs 1565–6, p. 65.

26. Cited in *NCOAP R & P*, 1 December 1923, p. 2; 18 October 1924, p. 4.

27. Wilson and Mackay, op. cit. p. 85.

28. *House of Commons Debates*, 5s, Vol. 184, 18 May 1925, Col. 90.

29. *PP* 1919, op. cit., *Minutes of Evidence*, Q. 1565, p. 65.

30. Paul Johnson, 'Self-help versus state-help: old age pensions and personal savings in Great Britain, 1906–1937', *Explorations in Economic History* (October 1984): 329–50; *Saving and Spending. The Working-Class Economy in Britain, 1870–1939*, Oxford: Oxford University Press, 1985, pp. 207–9, 215. A significant phenomenon of the inter-war years was the marked growth in the share of working-class funds invested in industrial assurance companies.

31. *NCOAP R & P*, 21 November 1925, p. 3; 16 May 1925, p. 6; *Review of Ten Years' Progress* (n.d. [1927], pp. 3–4.

32. *PP* 1919, op. cit., Q. 1112, p. 49.

33. Political and Economic Planning Memorandum, *Bournemouth Conservative Conference: Retirement Pensions*(7 October 1935), PEP Archives, WG 14/2.

34. *House of Commons Debates*, 5s, Vol. 184, 18 May 1925, Col. 100.

35. Social Insurance Committee (42) 9th Meeting, 6 May 1942, PRO CAB 87/77; S.I.C. (42) 11th Meeting: Part 1: *Minutes of 20 May 1942*, ibid.; 'Memorandum of Evidence by the National Federation of Old Age Pensions Associations', Social Insurance and Allied Services, Appendix G, Memoranda from Organisations, Cmd. 6405 (1942), p. 239.

36. Robert Skidelsky , *Oswald Mosley*, London: Macmillan, 1975, pp. 184–6.

37. Ernest Bevin, *My Plan for 2,000,000 Workless*, London: The Clarion Press, c. 1933.

38. *House of Commons Debates*, 5s, Vol. 286, 21 February 1934, Cols 419–73.

39. Political and Economic Planning, *The Exit from Industry*, London: PEP, 1935. There exists a large number of background papers to this report in the PEP Archives, British Library of Political and Economic Science. For PEP's origins, see John Pinder (ed.), *Fifty Years of Political and Economic Planning*, London: Heinemann, 1981.

40. *The Pensioner*, February 1940; March 1940; April 1940; May 1940; February 1941. It was reported in September 1940 that the Leith branch had begun as far back as 1929, but 'for many years made little progress'.

41. *The Pensioner*, September 1940; March 1941; June 1942; August 1942; May 1944; November 1942. In Autunn 1940, following hostilities on the National Council, the Northern Division of the National OAPA hived off to form the NFOAPA, with membership open to branches throughout the

country. The split proved anything but damaging to the growth of the movement.

42. *The Pensioner*, February 1940; J. Longstaff Dennison, *Plain Facts. Old Age Pensions As They Are and As They Ought To Be* (n.d., [c. 1919], p. 1.
43. *The Pensioner*, October 1942.
44. *The Pensioner*, January 1943.
45. J.C. Birtles, *The Ties That Bind* (n.d., unpaginated); *The Pensioner*, August 1943; May 1944.
46. Robin Means and Randall Smith, *The Development of Welfare Services for Elderly People*, London: Croom Helm, 1985, pp. 69-70.
47. The Pensioner, April 1940; October 1942; March 1942; September 1942; March 1940; April 1940; February 1940.
48. *The Pensioner*, February 1941.
49. *The Pensioner*, March 1941; April 1941; September 1941; December 1941; May 1941.
50. *The Pensioner*, August 1943, NFOAPA, Blackburn, local press cuttings and campaign leaflets, 1945.
51. Dan Carradice and Claude Stanfield, *Justice for the Old Folk*, London: ILP, 1943; *The Pensioner*, September 1943 — reprint of article by John McNair from *The New Leader*; *The Pensioner*, September 1942; May 1944; February 1945; September 1946; October 1984.
52. The National Council of Social Service, *The Needs of the Aged* (2 April 1942), PRO CAB 87/79. Where the National Council talked of 'problems of old people', Beveridge in his Report discussed 'the problem of age'.
53. S.I.C. (42) 1st Meeting, 14 January 1942, PRO CAB 87/77.
54. S.I.C. (42) 5th Meeting, 11 March 1942. ibid.
55. S.I.C. (42) 20: *Basic Problems of Social Security with Heads of a Scheme: Memorandum by the Chairman* (January 1942), PRO CAB 87/76.
56. S.I.C. (42) 1st Meeting, 14 January 1942, PRO Cab 87/77.
57. S.I.C. (42) 9th Meeting: Part 1, 6th May 1942, ibid.
58. Phillipson, op. cit., p. 29.
59. *Social Insurance and Allied Services* (Beveridge Report), Cmd. 6404, (1942), p. 91.
60. Ibid., p. 92.
61. Ibid., pp. 94-5.
62. Ibid., pp. 95-6.
63. Ibid., p. 96.
64. Ibid., p. 98.
65. S.I.C. (42) 136, *The Problem of Age: Memorandum by the Chairman* (20 August 1942), PRO CAB 87/82.
66. Means and Smith, op. cit., p. 70.
67. *The Pensioner*, January 1943; February 1943; May 1942.
68. For a preliminary investigation, see Stuart M.Riddle, 'Age, obsolesence and unemployment. Older men in the British industrial system, 1920-1939: a research note', *Ageing and Society* (December 1984): 517-24.
69. Noreen Branson and Margot Heinemann, *Britain in the Nineteen Thirties*, London: Weidenfeld and Nicolson, 1971, p. 226-7.

The Politics of Retirement, 1908–1948

Acknowledgements

We wish to acknowledge the support of the Economic and Social Research
Council, under whose grant (no. G01 250016) this research was conducted. For
allowing access to archive material, we should also like to thank the NFOAPA
(Headquarters, Melling House, Blackburn) and the British Library of Political
and Economic Science (PEP Archives). Crown copyright material in the Public
Record Office appears by permission of the Controller of Her Majesty's Stationery
Office.

© J hn Macnicol and Andrew Blaikie

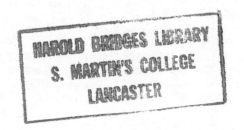

Chapter two

The Consolidation of 'Old Age' as a Phase of Life, 1945–1965[†]

Sarah Harper and Pat Thane

The social construction of old age in post-war Britain

This chapter focuses upon the post-war retirement debate. The decades following the Second World War saw an historically unprecedented growth in retirement at a fixed age for all social classes. The accompanying debate about population problems gave rise to much published discussion and research which reveals both the experiences and societal perceptions of the elderly in this period. It involved (not always successful) conscious efforts by influential groups and individuals to redefine the roles and popular images of elderly people.

Post-war Britain offers a suitable period in which to apply the concept of the social construction of old age. Whilst 'the elderly' have long been recognized as a distinct social category, ever-stricter stratification by age has emerged since industrialization (Thomas 1976; Quadragno 1982). This process has accelerated in the twentieth century and, we argue, reached completion in the twenty years following the Second World War. It entailed the increasing separation of biological from socially defined old age. In the post-war period, more universally than before, old age, and the socially accepted roles associated with it, was accepted as beginning at a fixed chronological age: the state pensionable age of 60/65.

'Retirement' provides an especially good opportunity to analyse this process. At earlier times, the move from full-time work to full-time retirement, through a transitional process of gradual movement of individuals through lighter and part-time employment, typically coincided with the biological transition from fitness to dependency. In recent times, however, most people have come to experience and to expect an *abrupt* transition from full-time work to full-time retirement at an age when many of them feel reasonably fit. This experience, which spread at an unusually fast pace in our period, especially among manual workers,

[†] This chapter is a shortened version of a longer paper, the full version of which can be obtained from the authors on request.

required adjustment on the part of individuals and society.

Taking a longer-term perspective it is also apparent that, during the post-war period from 1946 to the early 1960s, political, social, and economic changes combined to create a particular, historically new set of experiences and definitions of old age. Thus, for example, these decades saw the development of new services associated with the emerging welfare state and the expansion of state pensions to cover almost the entire elderly population. Also, the demographic structure was gradually shifting towards a higher representation of older age-groups (12 per cent aged 65 years or over in 1951, compared with 3.5 per cent in 1901), and changes in household composition produced increasing numbers of elderly people living alone (Wall 1982). Geriatrics became a serious medical specialty for the first time. Wartime discoveries of acute poverty among elderly people heightened awareness of their propensity to poverty.

These and other factors combined to give the elderly population a new and high profile in post-war public debate and social research. In particular, concern about the long-run decline in the birth-rate and the recognition that this was the major reason for the growing proportion of old people in the population (Thane forthcoming) coincided with a post-war labour shortage, making the elderly a focus of interest in a wider range of policy-making and otherwise influential circles. Issues concerning the elderly retained this high profile in social and economic research and in public debate until the early 1960s.

We argue that a specific set of widely held images of elderly people were constructed in this period. We have analysed processes behind this construction by examining the publications of academic, governmental and other public bodies, and of the mass media, remembering the cultural, political, and ideological context in which they were produced. These include the work of academic gerontologists, including industrial gerontologists, socio-medical geriatricians, social work specialists and sociologists; Hansard, the reports of government committees and other official publications; data from trade unions, business firms, political organizations, and pressure groups.

Concepts and Methods

Before considering the images of old age produced by such material, the concept of social construction itself requires brief discussion, as does the methodology employed. We have used the concept to mean the processes whereby specific social groups, in our case elderly people, come to be defined and categorized, and have characteristics attributed to them, which then become normative.

As regards methods of analysis, it seemed most appropriate to examine the output of selected key bodies, in order to make an assessment of the images of the elderly emerging from each and of similarities and differences among them. The bodies fell into a number of groups: social researchers, political representatives, the medical profession, and the organs of the mass media. The most problematic of these, in view of their diversity, were the first and the last. Ordering and analysing the output of the mass media obviously pose particular problems. Our approach in this case was to select specific events concerning the elderly, for example, the implementation of the new post-war pensions, the publication of official reports and of widely noticed social surveys, across the twenty-year time-span, and to review their presentation by newspapers and more specialized publications.

Research on the Elderly, 1945–65

The academic writing and research on old age from the late 1940s to the 1960s included studies of old people's economic circumstances, social networks, welfare and service provision, and residential circumstances, diet, socio-medical problems, and mental health. The research was funded from a wide variety of sources. There were four broad foci of research attention: employment, housing, social issues such as poverty and loneliness, and socio-medical issues.

While the research relating to the employment and retirement of older workers, as we shall see later, presented them in a positive light as net contributors to economy and society, the image emerging from other areas of analysis was more negative. Two broad themes were apparent: first, there was a growing recognition that elderly people were mentally and physically capable of far more than had been previously assumed, and that it was medically and socially possible for them to maintain an independent and active life. Running concurrent with this, however, was a belief that the community in the post-war period did little to ensure or support such life styles.

Medical research led the way in fostering the belief both in individual capacity and in community responsibiity for it. Until such pioneers as Marjorie Warren began to demonstrate otherwise in the 1930s, it was assumed that victims of strokes, for example, were incapable of rehabilitation. By 1948, however, Cosin was pointing out that the idea that most elderly patients were untreatable was a misconception. Accurate medical and social assessment, followed by treatment, could enable such patients to return to the community. It was this recognition that produced advances in geriatric medicine and ultimately a specialty provision in the NHS.

Such research tended to transfer the focus from elderly people themselves to their environment. Sheldon, in particular, demonstrated the close connection between social conditions and health (Sheldon 1948). This was followed by a series of studies of the relationship between living environments, the elderly, and ill health (Exton-Smith 1955), and of methods of minimizing length of stay in hospital by the establishment of out-patient assessment and follow-up clinics (Adams *et al* 1957), day hospitals (Cosin 1954), and preventive health care (Anderson and Cowan 1955).

The theme of the developing specialty of geriatrics was clear. Not only were the chronologically old (i.e. those over 60/65) capable of remaining within the community until biological old age was reached, but even then, given appropriate community support, many of them could enjoy a full personal and community life.

Social researchers and housing specialists produced a similar picture. They stressed that older people preferred to live independently both in their own houses and after admission to residential care and that this was possible if they were supported by kin and the wider community.

Despite this outpouring of research findings and recommendations, however, it appears that the immediate environment for the elderly changed very little during the period (Rowntree 1947; Utting 1958; Townsend 1962; Philips Committee — HMSO 1954). Indeed, Utting revealed that a fifth of the elderly population was at or below official subsistence level. There also remained throughout the period a general shortage of appropriate housing — in particular, a lack of accommodation for the frail and those with special needs (Townsend 1962; Webb 1962). None of this was surprising, since provision for elderly people represented an entirely new departure in house building.

In summary, the image created by the research of the period was of a growing sector of the population, able to remain active in the community after withdrawal from full-time paid labour, but only with the assistance of that community. Moreover, the need for assistance increased with age. The need to channel economic and social resources to the elderly population thus helped to present its image as a 'burden' on the community. Furthermore, the growing tendency to withdraw from economic activity at a specific chronological age (60/65), regardless of physiological condition and cognitive capacity, reinforced the attention paid to the ageing demographic structure of the country. The understandable concentration of research on the needy and on the failures of community support meant that little attention was paid to the *positive* contribution to the community made by many older people in the form of services to family and community.

Two further points about the research require emphasis. First, the research relating to employment focused almost entirely upon men (with the exception of Le Gros Clark 1962), whilst that into medical and social conditions studied mainly women. The different foci reflected the fact that the full-time paid labour force at retiring age was overwhelmingly male, whilst the majority of old people was female. Second, the two broad types of research focused on different age-groups. The labour force/retirement research focused on the 60–70 age-group, indeed sometimes drawing in those in their fifties, while the social research was more often concerned with those who were older and more dependent.

The retirement debate

Data from the 1931 to 1961 Censuses and from the Ministry of Social Security for 1966 showed a continuous decline in the percentage of men over the age of 65 in full-time paid employment (Table 2.1). The shift between 1931 and 1951 is particularly significant, since the former census was taken during a period of heavy unemployment when employment opportunities for older workers were at a low level and public opinion did not favour efforts to promote it; whilst in 1951 the exact opposite conditions prevailed.

Table 2.1 Percentage of age-group retired from full-time economic employment (males) (%)

Age	1931	1951	1961	1966
60–64	10.8	10.3	9.0	—
65–69	32.0	48.8	60.3	62.7
Over 70	63.3	77.1	88.7	—

Source: Census 1931, 1951, 1961; Ministry of Social Security, 1966.

Neither the Beveridge Report nor the National Insurance Act 1946 intended state-pension provision unnecessarily to remove able elderly workers from the labour market. Warning against encouraging the spread of early retirement, Beveridge recommended a system of increased pension rates as an incentive to defer retirement. The earnings allowance under the 1948 Act, which entitled those over 60/65 eligible for a contributory pension to earn a small amount without incurring deductions from their pension, was intended to discourage retirement at the minimum age (Hansard, Vol. 432, No. 150, Cols 1380–1472). Higher pensions were payable to those who remained in work beyond this age; these rose by annual increments for all retiring up to the age of 65/70. However, the level of both permissible earnings and of increments on deferment was too low to provide a significant disincentive to retirement — an indication of the Labour government's ambivalence on the issue. In contrast, the pension systems introduced in most other Western European countries facilitated flexible retirement ages by establishing a relationship on sliding scales between earnings and pensions. The reasons why this alternative was not adopted in Britain require investigation.

Political attitudes

The picture painted by these figures drew a response from various political and social bodies. Historically, the labour movement had been committed to earlier rather than later retirement. The Labour Party's pre-war proposals for improved old age pensions had included a retirement qualification. It had argued that adequate pension support for the elderly would encourage them to retire and thus increase younger workers' employment prospects. The Party experienced considerable problems in adjusting its policy to one of delaying retirement. However, during the Labour Government's first period of office, 1945–50, both the Ministry of Labour (through dissemination of information to employers) and the Ministry of National Insurance (through slightly increasing the earnings allowance) attempted to encourage the deferment of retirement beyond 65 and the employment of older workers.

Following their election in 1951, the Conservatives, who in principle were less fettered than the Labour Party since they possessed no traditional commitment to early retirement, introduced a more flexible retirement policy for civil servants. In 1953, the Ministry of Labour and National Service issued a memorandum on the Employment of Older Men and Women which claimed that 'for compelling social and economic reasons the door must be opened widely to the employment of people able and willing to work, irrespective of their age'. The memorandum (endorsed by the National Joint Advisory Council representing the British Employers' Confederation, the TUC, and the nationalized industries) identified as the essential problem the provision of a place in society for the ever-growing proportion of elderly persons and suggested that: 'Age sixty-five for men and sixty for women ought no longer to be regarded as "normal retiring age" '.

Appealing to employers to make special provision to enable older people to continue or, indeed, return to employment, the Ministry offered the help of its industrial rehabilitation units in cases where lack of confidence and low morale were obstacles to the re-employment of older people. It then established the National Advisory Committee on the Employment of Older Men and Women (Watkinson Committee). The Committee, however, in the first of its two reports in 1953 admitted that, despite isolated adjustments, no general or widespread changes had yet been made (HMSO 1953). Strongly opposing the maintenance of an essentially arbitrary general retirement-age, the Committee recommended that the test for engagement or retirement should be capacity, not age, and that all who could give effective service should have the chance to continue in work if they so wished.

The Second Report in 1955 (HMSO 1955) was more optimistic, with the Committee stating that its earlier recommendations had had some influence over employers. However, it recognized that 'the changes in employers' practices are to some extent due to acute labour shortages, particularly in some industrial areas'. Early in 1959 the Watkinson Committee was replaced by an interdepartmental committee assigned to co-ordinate research on the employment of older men and women. This was itself dissolved two years later. However, as the National Old People's Welfare Committee noted (1963:6), 'Since then there has been no apparent official action to promote the employment of elderly people'.

The Trades Unions

The Trades Union Congress stated generally that it had 'no firm views' on the 'problem of retirement'. However, two main objectives remained central to the movement throughout the period: early retirement combined with adequate state pensions.

Manual workers made up a large proportion of the TUC membership, and the health of many of these was depicted as having been destroyed by their employment; and, moreover, it was held that all workers had a right to a period of leisure in later life supported by a full subsistence pension. Early retirement had also long been advocated as a means of cutting unemployment and of encouraging the promotion of younger workers. Even during this period of labour shortage the fear of unemployment was ever present and remained a reality in certain occupations and regions, for example on Merseyside and Clydeside. It was understandably difficult for those whose views had been formed in a period of high unemployment to shift them radically and swiftly. The principle of the 'right to work' was extended to 'the right to work for all adults irrespective of age'; but it applied only where the labour of older workers was needed *in addition* to the full employment of younger men with families (Roberts 1954; Green 1963).

The TUC was also concerned that the retention of older workers would block promotion and thus the wage increments of the young (Green 1963). The TUC representatives on the Philips Committee issued a minority report opposing the Committee's recommendation to raise the minimum pension-age (TUC 1957:141). In addition, they supported the principle that receipt of the National Insurance pension should be conditional on retirement, because they feared that employers would treat pensions as a subsidy for wages if they were paid automatically at the age of 65 (ibid.). They thus called for a managerial policy to facilitate promotion earlier in life, linked to flexible retirement wherever possible.

At the same time, the unions gradually dropped their pre-war opposition to occupational pensions, recognizing the contribution they could make to their strategy of removing older workers from the labour market (Hannah 1986). It is apparent that the influence of the trades unions was highly significant, both at the level of negotiations with individual employers and through their influence on government policy.

Social research

Much of the post-war rise in social research into ageing and employment was under the auspices of the Nuffield Foundation. The Foundation's Annual Report for 1946 outlined its policy on the aged poor: 'As machines replace muscles as the motive force, the possibilities of extending useful employment could bring new purpose and new hope to those who have reluctantly accustomed themselves to being a burden' (p. 47) In that year the Foundation founded the Nuffield Research Unit into Problems of Ageing, at the University of Cambridge, with the purpose of studying 'those changes of human performance in middle and old age likely to have a bearing upon capacity for work in industry' (Nuffield Foundation 1953b: 160), a ten-year project. This was followed by grants (1954) to Murrell at Bristol. (Nuffield Foundation 1957: 87); to Szafran at Exeter (Nuffield Foundation 1958: 89); and to Le Gros Clark (Nuffield Foundation 1953a). During the 1950s further units were set up at London and Liverpool University to assess attitudes in industry.

The Foundation's concern with employment and the aged was also furthered by the establishment in 1947 of the National Corporation for the Care of Old People (Nuffield Foundation 1951). *Inter alia*, the NCCOP was concerned with problems arising from the community's attitudes to retirement (Nuffield Foundation, 1949).

The Debate

The retirement debate of the immediate post-war years was thus stimulated by a general awareness of the ageing of the population as a whole and of its work-force. Considerable alarm was expressed at these demographic changes (Thane forthcoming) although it was apparent that there was little idea of the possible economic and social implications. It must be noted, however, that although the work-force was ageing overall, not all sectors of industry were equally affected. In the early 1950s, males over 65 made up 3.3 per cent of the total manufacturing work-force, but they were 4.1 per cent in shipbuilding, 5.9 per cent in cotton spinning, 5.9 per cent in cotton weaving, 10.9 per cent in lace textiles, only 2 per cent in motor-vehicle manufacture. That is, they were more highly concentrated in the older staple industries which were in acute and widely recognized need of restructuring, the labour shortage was most acute in some of the highly skilled sectors of these very industries, and their loss would be acutely felt, at least in the short term. Hence, although older workers did not contribute a large proportion of the work-force, their placing in the economy and the nature of the post-war economic problem made contemporary concern about them understandable. Of greater long-term importance was the fact that the *entire* work-force was shifting in its age structure towards later ages.

Realization of how little was known about the likely effects of this demographic change led to the production of the first substantial body of data in this country on the experience of ageing in industry and on the relationship of work capacity to ageing: a highly polemical debate received some empirical clothing. Three broad streams of concern were apparent — over the national economy, over individual health and personal welfare, and over the moral obligations of society to its older citizens. It was the first two which carried most force and were backed by the most extensive social research.

The National Economy: the Dependency Argument

The stance most widely adopted by politicians, demographers, and economists was closely related to some of the eugenist arguments of the inter-war years: namely that the ageing of the population would create an unbalanced ratio of workers to dependents, with severe social and economic consequences. As a consequence of the belief in the unbalanced ratio, demographers advocated the long-term necessity of keeping older people in the work-force, since the birth-rate was expected to remain low despite a wartime upturn.

The Philips Report (HMSO 1954) forecast little change in the dependency ratio overall in the following twenty-five years (1954–79), on the assumption that the same proportion of persons would continue to be employed in each age-group. In doing so it used the temporary 1951–3 increase in employment of older workers rather than the *wider post-war* trend to earlier retirement. Nevertheless, the Report estimated that the *proportion* of dependents who were elderly would increase over that period from 12 per cent to nearly a third by 1979.

Fears were thus expressed that, while the ratio of all dependents to the total population might be no greater in the immediate future than in the past, the cost per dependent had grown and would continue to grow. Parish and Peacock (1954) calculated that twice as much was spent per capita by the five major social services on pensioners as on children, and three-and-a-half times as much as on the active population. Similarly, Shenfield, relying entirely upon Parish and Peacock for her calculations, asserted that while the number of old people rose by two-and-a-half times between 1910 and 1954, the proportion of the national income transferred to the elderly during the same period had quadrupled (Shenfield 1957).

The polemical and ideological edge to this debate must be borne in mind: not all those engaged in it were in favour of increased public spending, due to fears about its effects on investment and on incentives; and in some quarters it was passionately felt that the ageing of society was socially, economically, and even politically undesirable (Thane forthcoming), and hence that its dangers should be emphasized. In fact, no calculations were published which attempted to measure the precise costs or specify the benefits to be derived from an ageing population. The emphasis was on the burden of cost unpaid by the elderly.

The employment of older workers was seen as tackling the dependency problem from two angles. The first was the view that such workers would make a positive contribution to the national economy and directly ease the labour shortage. However, as the Philips Report (HMSO 1954) pointed out: 'The contribution to be expected from any likely postponement of retirement would not appear to be large in relation to total available manpower.'

The other argument for encouraging prolonged economic activity was that it would relieve the financial burden on the Exchequer of the cost of pensions and services to the elderly population. While accepting that if national productivity increased at the then current rate and priority in the allocation of social expenditure was given to the elderly, the current pension-policies could be maintained, the Philips Committee stressed the magnitude of the commitments being entered into on behalf of future generations of taxpayers. Similarly, the Government Actuary reported that current expenditure on retirement pensions was already higher than that part of the insurance contribution assigned for the purpose (HMSO 1954: para. 161).

The Philips Report was so concerned about the increasing proportion of elderly people in the population that it thought some rise in the minimum pension-age inevitable. It thus recommended that the age should ultimately be raised to 68 for men and 63 for women.

The second strand of the economic argument was the suggestion that industry would positively benefit from the encouragement, retention, and retraining of elderly workers. Welford (1953) was a keen protagonist of this argument.

Ageing and work capacity — the arguments

Welford's Cambridge group set out to identify the nature of the work for which the older worker was best suited and the most suitable methods of retraining those whose skills had become redundant as the result of modifications in the industrial process (Welford 1951). Its main conclusions were that while there were major changes in capacity with age, in particular in mental capacity, which affected the employability of an individual, these could all be overcome to varying degrees by an alteration in the work environment. While loss of learning ability among the elderly appeared primarily linked to difficulties in understanding, recall, and error abandonment, if these were corrected at an early stage 'old people can learn much more readily than is commonly supposed' (Welford 1966: 5). The research also demonstrated that older workers could maximize their efficiency if they were able to control their own work pace. Hence they could cope better with heavy manual labour, which allowed them to pause when they chose, than with continuous process work, both of the latter being growing trends in industry.

Le Gros Clark approached the problem from the angle of the work environment. Arguing that machines must be adapted to men, rather than men to machines, he was one of the first to recognize the importance of a versatile work-force, adjusted from an early age to job transference in later life, within a flexible environment which allowed movement between jobs (Le Gros Clark 1954b).

Health and personal welfare — the arguments

The second group of arguments in the retirement debate concerned the health and welfare of the older individual. The image presented was of potentially active individuals bereft both of health and satisfaction through enforced retirement from economic activity.

The 'retirement impact hypothesis' (McMahon and Ford 1955) — the suggestion that retirement leads to ill health or even death having been out of favour during the inter-war depression (Emerson 1959) was resurrected during the post-war period. Support by members of the medical profession made it particularly attractive. While this hypothesis was systematically studied in the USA, British research specifically into this area was neglible. One or two surveys revealed better health and a greater degree of satisfaction among the occupied over pension age than among the retired (Anderson and Cowan 1955; Welford 1966), and the high death-rate in the first year following cessation of work was often quoted to prove that retirement might speed premature deterioration.

With the exception of certain areas of mental health, there appeared little clear medical evidence in support of these claims. The debate appears to have been conducted in some ignorance but, as with much else in this area, a high degree of polemical certitude. The compulsory retirement of active, healthy elderly people who were willing to continue working was seen as a contributory factor to the high rate of suicide among the aged (WHO 1959; Logan 1953) which peaked at age 70; deferred retirement was advocated as a preventive measure (Batchelor and Napier 1953). There appeared to be limited evidence that some sleep disorders might be connected with sudden retirement (Cowan 1956)

53

and that disability and senility might be delayed through the prolonging of an active working life (Thompson 1949; Shenfield 1963). Beyond this, however, many of the claims were supported by anecdotal and subjective impressions only.

One exception was the work of Emerson, based at the University of Nottingham. Pointing out the pitfalls of much of the past research, he drew on his study of 125 65-year-old men to argue that those who had recently retired were a 'transitional' group between those still in full-time employment and those settled into retirement (Emerson 1959). The tensions that did arise were generated during the period of readjustment and later resolved. Furthermore, his study suggested that, even during the first, 'transitional' year, retirement *per se* had little effect on physical or mental health. Too much research based conclusions on too short a time-scale.

The retirement impact hypothesis appeared to spread quickly and to be widely accepted, particularly in governmental and other widely disseminated documents.

The image and the wider community

The image produced within both the political and the socio-medical arena was forceful. It was that a significant proportion of the elderly population was an asset to the community if allowed to be economically active, but a burden, both to itself and to society, if forced to retire.

The aged as an economic asset

The economic component of the image was clearly aimed at employers, in particular in industry. Contemporary surveys indicate that industry was either unaware of this component of the debate or chose to disregard it. Indeed, a major theme which emerged at this time was the lack of attention given by employers to the age structure of their work-forces and the consequent lack of encouragement to older people to see themselves as potentially economically viable.

A survey in 1951 of the 400 member firms of the Industrial Welfare Society revealed that they had not attempted to consider, let alone assess, the profitability of employing elderly workers (Industrial Welfare Society 1951). A similar picture was painted in Fleming's assessment (1955) of the iron and steel industry in 1952. Of even greater interest was Fleming's survey of the Sheffield cutlery industry in 1960 (1963). This revealed that the management were 'concerned' that the post-60/65 group comprised 18 per cent of the industry compared with a national average of 3.5 per cent, and had offered 'solutions'. However, not only had these been implemented by only a few firms, but the majority were also oriented towards encouraging youth employment rather than positive action to assist older workers. Heron and Chown concluded that 'Industry in general simply does not acknowledge a problem of ageing' (Heron and Chown 1961: 16). In practice, then, there appeared to be no general fixed set of expectations of behaviour towards elderly workers on the part of employers.

Shenfield's survey of the Midlands' manufacturing industry in 1954 (Shenfield 1957) revealed that over three-quarters of firms had flexible pension schemes, as did the analysis of the London County Council building trade (Le Gros Clark 1954a and b). However, the position towards the end of the decade appeared less clear.

Although policies obviously varied according to the occupational structure and size of the company (Hannah 1986), large organizations were considered more likely to instigate rigid retirement policies than were small ones (Acton Society Trust 1960). Increasing technology (Le Gros Clark 1968) and complicated administrative structures (Green 1963) were also likely to encourage rigid policies. The general trend appears to have been towards making it more difficult for people to stay on in full-time employment after 65 (Heron and Chown 1961).

The surveys also gave some indication of contemporary attitudes to elderly workers, although, bearing in mind the general lack of positive attention paid to such workers, it is necessary to treat the data with caution. Indeed, several of the researchers noted that their evidence was produced after the plight of the elderly had been drawn to the attention of employers, foremen, and co-workers (Shenfield 1957; Acton Society Trust 1960; Fleming 1963). The evidence is of both positive and negative reactions to the older worker as employee and co-worker.

The forties were seen as the age of potential transition from 'young' to 'old'. For example, a survey of just under 1,000 firms in the 1950s (Industrial Welfare Society 1951) found that, even among the employers of skilled workers, a third were doubtful as to the worth of those over 45, while 6 per cent considered such men 'too old'.

It is clear that many of these kinds of views were based on the evidence that in some areas of employment, and in particular on production lines involving speed and pacing, problems began as early as the mid to late forties. In industries already geared to fast-paced work, such as motor-vehicle manufacture, it is therefore not surprising that there was little interest in older workers. One of the problems of the Ministry of Labour was to reconcile demands for increased mechanization to promote productivity with demands that older workers be kept on. It was not therefore surprising that few industries had a positive policy of encouraging the employment of those past statutory retirement pension age.

The available survey material suggests that, while certain employers were prepared to retain individual workers beyond the official retirement age by virtue of their particular merits (Shenfield 1957), there was no determined effort by industry to accommodate elderly workers.

The conclusion is either that the political and social message concerning older workers was not reaching employers, whose strategies were determined by other priorities, or that they put the immediate interests of the firm, as they defined them, before the longer-term interest of the national economy as the government was defining it. Following a decade of political and socio-medical pressure to retain elderly employees, industrial management had still not given significant attention to the effective utilization of older workers. Fleming concluded that information relating to the elderly worker did not readily reach the attention of management (Fleming 1963).

The message appeared to have reached workers more quickly. Rose reported in 1953 that 79 per cent of a sample of unemployed older men in Hull knew 'that the country was asking people to stay on at work after retiring age' and 74 per cent of them thought this a 'reasonable thing' (Rose 1953). It seems reasonable to conclude that employers and managers were unlikely to have missed the message but had consciously rejected it.

The impact of retirement

While the concept of elderly people as constructive members of the workforce may have failed to influence industry, the idea that retirement led to death and deterioration appeared to have been widely established. Emerson revealed that both those who continued working and those who retired 'appeared to be to some extent affected by rather garbled information concerning retirement impact' (Emerson 1959). Other studies reported fear among workers that the cessation of employment would lead to a rapid deterioraton in health and mobility (Townsend 1955; Groombridge 1960; Nuffield Foundation 1963). Townsend noted a preconceived association between retirement, ill health and death within the wider community which may have had older cultural roots.

It was an image disseminated by the media. While it is not possible to determine how widespread it was, examples were found in specialized journals and publications for the wider public. An article in the *Nursing Times* of 23 August 1957, for example, stressed the importance of work as a cure for the ills of old age (pp. 945–6), followed four months later by one in the *Nursing Mirror*: 'Occupation is unquestionably one of the most important factors in preserving mental alertness and bodily health.' (10 January 1958 p. 1)

Social services personnel were also quick to take up the theme. In

1953, the British National Conference on Social Work warned of the problems of abrupt retirement, while throughout the decade old people's welfare committees acted to find work for the elderly. In 1951, the Employment Fellowship (formerly the Winter Distress League) turned to the problem of keeping elderly people employed for as long as possible (Employment Fellowship 1958). In co-operation with Finsbury Borough Council it established the first 'sheltered' work-room where 'elderly workers could be employed for two hours a day, on small assembling and packing jobs provided by local firms, paying the fair rate for the work completed'.

On similar lines the NOPWC reported in 1963 that some nineteen employment agencies were being run by old people's welfare committees 'to give older workers the opportunity to continue working beyond retirement age' and prevent them 'being thrown on a human scrap heap where their physical and mental health suffered and some became prematurely incapable of leading independent lives' (NOPWC 1963: 4).

Such schemes were an attempt to accommodate the desire of many older people to continue in at least part-time work and to find new ways of continuing the older tradition of gradual transition from full-time work to full retirement. Once again, employers showed little enthusiasm for them.

In 1955, the NOPWC appointed a study group to consider preparation for retirement, which resulted in the establishment of the Preparation for Retirement Committee in 1960. Its brief was to 'help and persuade as many people as possible to look forward to retirement as the time of fulfilment' (Hubbard 1962). The Committee called on industry, commerce, the education services, religious and statutory bodies, and voluntary organizations to aid it in its task. The following year both the Industrial Welfare Society and the Institute of Directors held conferences on retirement preparation, with the Preparation for Retirement Committee holding its first national conference in 1963. In 1960, the Acton Society Trust had reported being unaware of any company which had a programme of preparation for retirement. Over the next five years various publications advocating such courses were made available to industry. In 1962, the Institute of Directors (IOD) established a Retirement Advisory Bureau; and the first private retirement consultancy was set up in London in 1965 (IPM 1965). By then at least twenty major national and international companies had established pre-retirement schemes for their work-forces (ibid.), and seventeen pre-retirement associations/councils, now extant throughout the UK, ran courses and conferences for firms and the general public on retirement. Such schemes were generally directed at all employees, manual, white collar, and managerial, although the percentage of each section attending such courses is unclear.

A working party set up in 1966 by the Yorkshire Council of Social Services to study regional preparation for retirement (Yorkshire Council of Social Services 1966) reported an encouraging level of interest on the part of larger industrial enterprises, but a relative lack of concern in the retail trade, commerce, and smaller industrial units.

In summary

To summarize, two positive images of elderly people were created by the employment debate. The first defined them as potentially active and vital contributors to the economy; the second as vulnerable individuals who would be bereft of both health and personal satisfaction by enforced retirement. The first construction was not appropriated by employers. The second aroused more positive interest, though it is unclear with what precise effect. While the exact *relationship* between retirement and ill health was unclear, an *association* between the two was sufficiently apparent to result in apprehension being experienced by elderly workers and their families. Such beliefs, coinciding with the growing phenomenon of abrupt cessation of full-time employment, encouraged the growth of the preparation-for-retirement movement.

By the beginning of the 1960s the government had given up the attempt to encourage employers to take special note of the needs of older workers. In 1964, the annual *Labour Gazette* stopped printing annual retirement figures. Fears of a national labour shortage had eased and were replaced by fears of large-scale unemployment due to the spread of 'automation' (Bagrit 1965). The abolition of national service, Commonwealth immigration, the entry into the labour market of the 'baby boom' generation, and the increasing numbers of married women remaining in or returning to work all provided additional supplies of labour. To what extent they provided substitutable labour for older, skilled workers is another, unresearched, question; but, in general, interest in older workers as a source of labour and in the effects of their work and retirement status on their own health and that of the national economy waned.

Conclusion — image, context, and control

This discussion of the main elements of the retirement debate has demonstrated the ways in which the establishment of an image of a social group — the old — was linked into the specific conditions of an historical period. That part of the image which had the most resonance both with elderly workers and their employers was that of 'retirement impact' — that is, of the physical and mental ill effects assumed to be associated with retirement. Employers in general appeared to see ageing people as a national responsibilty rather than as their immediate concern.

A new tradition of retirement was thus consolidated during the period. During the 1950s and early 1960s, retirement at the statutory pensionable age of 60 for men and 65 for women became widely established across occupations and social classes, although least at the highest status-levels. By the late 1960s, it was accepted that the *normal* period of full-time economic employment would cease for *most* of the population at these ages.

Society gradually adjusted to the emergence of a new distinct phase in the life cycles of most people, a period of post-employment leisure normally preceding by many years the onset of marked physical decline. At the same time, however, no positive socially accepted role emerged for people experiencing this period. While society may have been identifying 'old age' as a distinct phase of life, it was providing little practical support for individuals experiencing it. It took a further two decades before 'the elderly' were once more to experience the high profile that they had achieved in the debates of the 1940s and 1950s concerning their position and role in the economy.

Acknowledgement

We wish to acknowledge the support of the ESRC under whose grant (no. GO125007) this research was conducted.

References

Published material

Acton Society Trust (1960) *Retirement: A Study of Current Attitudes and Practices*, London: Acton Society Trust.

Adams, G., McQuitty, F., and Flint, M. (1957) *Rehabilitation of the Elderly Invalid at Home*, Nuffield Provincial Hospitals Trust.

Anderson, W. and Cowan, N. (1955) *The Lancet* 2: 239.

Bagrit, L. (1965) *The BBC Reith Lectures, 1964: The Age of Automation*, London: Weidenfeld and Nicolson.

Batchelor, I. and Napier, M. (1953) *British Medical Journal* 2: 1186.

Cosin, L. (1948) *Proceedings, Royal Society of Medicine* 41.

Cosin, L. (1954) *The Practitioner*: 172.

Emerson, A. (1959) 'The first year of retirement', *Occupational Psychology* 34: 197–208.

Exton-Smith, A. (1955) *Medical Problems in Old Age*, Bristol: J. Wright & Sons.

Fleming, C. (1963) 'The age factor in the Sheffield cutlery industry', *Vita Humana* 6(4): 177–212.

Green, G. (1963) *The Trade Unions*, Preparation for Retirement First National

Conference, September.
Groombridge, B. (1960) Education and Retirement, The National Institute of Adult Education.
Hannah, L. (1986) *Inventing Retirement: The Development of Occupational Pensions in Great Britain*, Cambridge University Press.
HMSO (1953) *Employment of Older Men and Women*, Advisory Committee of the Ministry of Labour and National Service, First Report, Cmd. 8963.
HMSO (1954) *Report of the Committee on the Economic and Financial Problems of the Provision for Old Age* (The Philips Report), Cmd. 9333.
HMSO (1955) *Employment of Older Men and Women*. Advisory Committee of the Ministry of Labour and National Service, Second Report, Cmd. 9628.
Hubbard, L. (1962) 'The Preparation for Retirement Committee', *Society of Housing Managers Quarterly Journal* 5: 10–11.
Le Gros Clark, F. (1954a) *The Later Working Life in the Building Industry*, Nuffield Foundation.
Le Gros Clark, F. (1954b) *The Working Fitness of Older Men*, Nuffield Foundation.
Le Gros Clark, F. (1962) *Women, Work and Age*, Nuffield Foundation.
Logan, W. (1953) *British Medical Journal* 2: 1190.
McMahon, C. and Ford, T. (1955) 'Surviving the first five years of retirement', *Journal of Gerontology* 10: 212–15.
Parish, F. and Peacock, A. (1954) 'Economics of dependence', *Economica* 21: 84.
Quadragno, J. (1982) *Ageing in Early Industrial Society: Work, Family and Social Policy in Nineteenth Century England*, New York: Academic Press.
Rose, A.B. (1953) *The Older Unemployed Man in Hull*, University of Hull, Department of Social Studies paper: 14.
Sheldon, J. (1948) *The Social Medicine of Old Age*, Nuffield Foundation.
Shenfield, B. (1957) *Social Policies for Old Age*, London: Routledge & Kegan Paul.
Thane, P. (forthcoming) 'The debate on the declining birth rate and the 'menace' of an ageing population in Britain, 1930–1950'.
Thomas, K. (1976) 'Age and authority in early modern England', *Proceedings of the British Academy*, 62: 205–48
Thompson, A. (1949) 'Problems of ageing and chronic sickness': The Hunterian lectures, British Medical Journal 2: 263.
Townsend, P. (1955) 'The construction of retirement', *Transactions of the Association of Industrial Medical Officers* 5.
Townsend, P. (1962) 'The meaning of poverty', *British Journal of Sociology* 13(3): pp. 210–27.
Utting, J. (1958) *Survey of the Economic Circumstances of Old People in Great Britain*, Nuffield Foundation.
Wall, R. (1982) 'Regional and temporal variations in the structure of the British household since 1851', in T. Barker and M. Drake (eds), *Population and Society in Britain 1850–1980*, London: Batsford, pp. 62–99.
Webb, M. (1962) 'Housing societies to help the aged', *Society of Housing Managers Quarterly Journal* 5: 7–10.

Welford, A.T. (1951) *Skill and Age*, Oxford University Press for the Nuffield Foundation.

Welford, A.T. (1953) 'Extending the employment of older people', *British Medical Journal*, 1193–7.

Welford, A.T. (1966) 'Industrial work suitable for older people: some British studies', *Gerontologist*, 6 March: 4–9.

WHO (1959) *Mental Health Problems of Ageing and the Aged*, World Health Organization, Technical Report Series, no. 171.

Unpublished Material and Annual Reports

Cowan, N. (1956) 'Sleep Behaviour and the Aged', Health Bulletin, Department of Health for Scotland.

Employment Fellowship (1958) *Workrooms for the Elderly*.

Fleming, C. (1955) 'Ageing in an industry: an age-compositional investigation of workforces in the British iron and steel industry, 1952–3, mimeo, pp. 1–76.

Heron, A. and Chown, S. (1961) 'Ageing and the semi-skilled: a survey in manufacturing industry on Merseyside', *Med. Res. Council Mem.* 40: 1–49.

Industrial Welfare Society (1951) *The Employment of Elderly Workers*, IWS.

Institute of Personnel Management (1965) *Managing Retirement*, IPM.

National Old People's Welfare Committee (1963) *Employment and Workshops for the Elderly*, NOPWC.

Nuffield Foundation (1946) *Annual Report*, Oxford University Press.

Nuffield Foundation (1949) *Annual Report*, Oxford University Press.

Nuffield Foundation (1951) *Annual Report*, Oxford University Press.

Nuffield Foundation (1953a) *Annual Report*, Oxford University Press.

Nuffield Foundation (1953b) *Review of the First Ten Years, 1943–1953*, Oxford University Press.

Nuffield Foundation (1957) *Annual Report*, Oxford University Press.

Nuffield Foundation (1958) *Annual Report*, Oxford University Press.

Nuffield Foundation (1963) *Workers Nearing Retirement*, Nuffield Foundation.

Roberts, A. (1954) 'British Trade Union Attitudes to the Employment of Older Men and Women', Third Congress of the International Association of Gerontology.

Rowntree, B.S. (1947) *Old People: report of a survey committee on the problems of ageing and the care of old people*, Nuffield Foundation Oxford University Press.

Shenfield, B. (1963) 'Historical and demographic background', in *Preparation for Retirement*, NOPWC First National Conference, September, pp. 7–12.

TUC (1957) *Annual Report*.

Yorkshire Council of Social Services (1966) *Preparation for Retirement: A Regional Study*, YCSS.

© Sarah Harper and Pat Thane

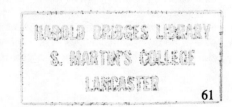

Chapter three

The Structured Dependency of the Elderly: A Critical Note[1]

Paul Johnson

Social gerontology draws on a broad range of social science disciplines for its theories and methodologies, but to date its debt to economics and economists has been slight. Aside from a passing interest in the impact of the State Earnings Related Pension Scheme on future tax burdens, economists seem generally to have ignored the issues of elderly people and of ageing. Economic questions have been left largely to social policy analysts to look at, and much of their writing has been placed squarely within a radical framework often described by the term 'the political economy of ageing'. Economic questions about ageing are seen by them to have an explicitly political dimension because the state, being the major determinant of the economic status of the elderly population, is regarded as capable (and culpable) of creating a new sort of deliberately structured dependency among old people.

This note challenges this particular thesis that has been developed most clearly in the writings of Peter Townsend, Alan Walker, and Chris Phillipson,[2] and suggests that concentration on the concept of structured dependency has deflected attention away from more progressive and optimistic views of the economic social status of the elderly in modern Britain.

In writings on the political economy of ageing, it has been suggested that twentieth-century society has deliberately promoted the marginalization and dependency of elderly people, and that the state has played a major role in this process. For instance, Townsend writes that: 'the concepts of retirement [and] pensionable status . . have been developed in both capitalist and state socialist countries in ways which have created and reinforced the social dependency of the elderly';[3] and Walker believes that: 'dependency at both ends of the age spectrum has been enlarged by social and economic developments over the course of this century'.[4] The argument that the dependent status of elderly people has been deliberately structured by the state and society takes the economic conditions of the non-institutionalized elderly as being at the root of their dependent status. The explicit or implicit argument is that elderly people have experienced a constriction of economic liberty in

62

modern Britain because of the sometimes deliberate and sometimes unconscious course of development of social welfare and employment policies. Much of the detailed research that has made use of the concept of structured dependency has, however, focused on the relatively small and exceptional subgroup of elderly people living in institutions, for whom the concept of dependency seems more immediately relevant,[5] and this may have biased the outlook of social policy analysts in their discussion of the much larger group of economically and socially independent elderly.

This chapter examines the broader economic circumstances of non-institutionalized elderly people, and the way these have changed over the last eighty years, to see how far and in what areas they may challenge the assertions of the 'structured dependency' school of authors.

Before doing so, some longer-run historical trends need to be mentioned briefly, because implicit in much of the writing on the social creation of dependency is the belief that elderly people were in many ways more independent in a pre-welfare state age. Townsend, for example, has written that 'such "structured" dependency is a consequence of twentieth-century thought and action'.[6] Historians such as Richard Smith and David Thomson, however, have shown how enduring and old-fashioned are many twentieth-century patterns of thought and action — such as retirement from the work-force in old age, and the provision of financial and other services for elderly people by the community rather than by kin.[7] Thomson has taken the issue further, arguing that many twentieth-century writers on social welfare issues have been misled into believing that recent developments represent an abrupt break with historical experience because of the peculiarly restrictive and individualistic support systems for elderly people that emerged in the late Victorian period.[8] This historical work itself represents a strong challenge to some of the premises which underpin the idea of structured dependency. However, the discussions of commentators like Townsend, Walker, and Phillipson focus primarily on twentieth-century developments, and it is on changes in the economic status of elderly people since 1900 that this chapter will concentrate.

The economic status of the elderly is, in outline, determined by four factors:

(1) their employment status;
(2) their access to state pensions and welfare benefits;
(3) their access to private savings (especially occupational) pensions; and
(4) their receipt of familial support.

Any attempt to determine either the direction of or the reason for changes in economic status must look at these four factors separately.

Since rising retirement rates among elderly people have been one of the striking developments in labour market behaviour this century, it seems appropriate to begin by looking at the reasons why the employment status of the elderly population has changed so much over time, and the consequences of this change.

Employment

In 1901, almost 60 per cent of the male population of England and Wales aged 65 and over was recorded in the census as occupied; the corresponding figure for women was 13.4 per cent. These occupational rates for the elderly were virtually constant across the 1911 and 1921 Censuses. They showed some decline in the 1931 Census (to 48 per cent and 8 per cent respectively), part of which must have been the result of high general levels of unemployment in the depths of the inter-war depression. The most rapid decline in employment among elderly people has come about since the Second World War, with the proportion of men over 65 in employment falling from 30 per cent to 10 per cent between 1951 and 1981, although, because of a rise in married women's employment, the proportion of the female population over 60 in employment was about the same in 1981 (8 per cent) as in 1951.[9]

These changes in the participation rates of the elderly must be due either to a reduction in the demand for the labour of this section of the population, or a reduction in the labour services offered or supplied by the elderly, or some combination of the two. Changes in these supply and demand factors depend on the physical and mental capacity of individuals for work and the requirements of employment, but also on the personal choice of individuals, the marginal productivity of other groups in the labour market, the flexibility of remuneration schemes, and institutional factors such as pension-scheme regulations. In much of the writing on the dependent elderly, the assumption has been made that retirement has become more common at an earlier age because of a reduction in the demand for elderly workers. Phillipson suggests that the elderly have been deliberately relegated to a reserve army of labour,[10] and Walker concurs: 'Retirement is a largely twentieth century phenomenon, which has been managed to remove from employment older workers in order to reconstitute and re-skill the labour force.'[11]

There are, however, no theoretical grounds for preferring demand-side explanations for the growth of retirement to supply-side ones, and the evidence available on changes in the retirement process in twentieth-century Britain is ambiguous. It is true that Hannah's work on occupational pension schemes suggests that large companies may have managed the retirement process in order to control their internal labour markets, but for most of the century such schemes have covered only a minority of workers.[12] Phillipson has pointed to more direct state management of retirement, in order to regulate the size of the labour force, yet the well-known attempts by the government to induce retirees back to work after the Second World War were notable for their lack of success; the reserve army of elderly labour was highly resistant to re-enlistment.[13]

It seems likely that improvements in the health and work capacity of the elderly population over the last eighty years have more than compensated for any putative increase in the physical and mental demands of employment; if so, rising retirement rates may reflect a decrease in the demand for the labour of elderly workers over a period in which their employment capacity has risen. The introduction by employers of fixed retirement-ages, frequently linked to the minimum age for the receipt of the state's retirement pension, is commonly viewed as an important demand-side influence, but the evidence is by no means conclusive. It is clear from data on occupations drawn from the decennial censuses that retirement for men over the age of 65 was increasing from 1881, almost thirty years before the introduction of a state pension; and modern evidence from the United States gives good grounds for believing that, in some circumstances at least, changes in retirement age over time represent a supply-side factor, with people choosing retirement before they become incapable of work. The 1978 Age Discrimination in Employment Act, which raised the minimum mandatory retirement age in the US from 65 to 70, was followed by a fall in the average age of retirement, and the option to choose retirement before 65 at a reduced pension is being taken by an increasing number of American workers.[14] In British writing on retirement, however, and particularly in the writing of the radical 'structured dependency' school, supply-side factors — i.e. the desires of workers — have played a muted second fiddle to demand-side analysis.

There are two reasons for the emphasis on demand, and they both relate to some of the premises built into the idea of 'structured dependency'. The first is that, despite their radical appearance, ideas of structured dependency or 'the social construction of old age dependency' have their origins in functionalist social-control theories. They therefore stress the coherence of the views and power of the controlling group (usually 'the state' or 'capitalism'), and pay little attention to the responses of the group being controlled, in this case elderly people, who are assumed to have little if any room for manœuvre. Exactly how the controlling group agrees on common interests and actions is not specified, though the implication is of some quasi-conspiratorial corporatist process. (Hannah's work on occupational pensions suggests that employers could seldom conspire, because they seldom had any idea of what they were doing in the area of pension policy.) In addition, why the controlled group chooses to be compliant, or why it may choose to be resistant to any process of control, is also ignored. Indeed, the very idea of resistance is generally excluded from social-control theories, because the deviant group is perceived to be powerless, forever the object of someone else's control, never the subject of its own thoughts and actions. The intellectual origins of structured dependency ideas in functionalist social-control theories inevitably focuses attention on employers and the state, and diminishes the importance of choice exercised by elderly people themselves.

The second reason why the desires of workers are underemphasized in 'structured dependency' writings is the acceptance of the thoroughly capitalist convention that worth is determined primarily by participation in the productive process. There is an explicit belief in the literature that the transition from independent to dependent status comes on retirement. Because retirement creates dependency, and dependency is undesirable, retirement is unlikely to be chosen voluntarily; therefore the study of retirement has to focus on labour demand from employers, not labour supply from workers.

However, this line of argument is hardly what radical analysts of the welfare state should want. It suggests that a 65 year-old retiree with a large private income is in some meaningful sense more dependent than a 64 year-old labourer in receipt of a low weekly wage. Alan Walker acknowledges a difficulty here when he writes:

> The fact that many workers in these societies are themselves *dependent* on the owners of capital for the hire of their labour power is one of the factors that would be included in a more considered analysis of this link [between dependency and production],[15]

but he then goes on to ignore it. As long as those who use the concept of structured dependency continue to make the automatic association of retirement with dependency, and of work with independence, they will continue to bolster conservative notions of the competitive work ethic. The reason they do this is in order to link general criticisms of the capitalist economic system with a specific analysis of the poverty of the elderly, but in doing so they shift their point of reference. The dependency that they believe results from retirement stems from an inability to produce, but poverty stems from an inability to consume. In a world with saving and intergenerational transfers, marginalization in production need not be equated with marginalization in consumption, and any extension of savings or transfers must tend to lessen the importance of employment status in establishing overall economic status. If it is accepted that ability to consume is the major determinant and indicator of economic status — and that is implicit in the common concern over the 'standard of living' of different groups in society — then the conclusion must be that retirement is only one of a number of factors that affect economic status, and retirement alone is neither a necessary nor a sufficient condition for economic dependency. If retirement does not inevitably involve economic dependency, then it is easy to see how retirement may result from a positive choice by those people who believe they will not suffer any substantially reduced ability to consume.

Of course, people do not work simply for economic rewards, and there may be other social and psychological losses on retirement (though equally there may be gains). It is, however, the financial losses of retirement from the labour force that seem usually to be taken as the key to the involuntary shift from independence to dependency in old age. By defining retirement as coterminous with dependency, the 'structured dependency' authors inevitably see the trend towards earlier retirement as regrettable, but in fact it need not be so: this depends on the extent to which retirement leads subsequently to poverty in old age, and to discover this it is necessary to look at the other three main determinants of the financial status of the elderly.

State benefits

The rise in the importance of state benefits in the financial status of elderly people over the course of this century is something noted by virtually all commentators, though it should be remembered that many elderly people relied on Poor Law support before the payment of state old-age pensions in 1909. This expansion of the role of the state has variously been interpreted as a functional response to old age incapacity, an indication of the growing humanity of welfare capitalism, or, by radical analysts, as part of a deliberate attempt to reconcile elderly people to a status of dependency. Again it seems that the radical critique has confused form and content, and so has directed valuable criticisms about the level of state support towards the form of state support itself.

There is no theoretical reason to suppose that a transition from labour market income to state benefit income induces the onset of dependency: indeed, logically the reverse should happen, as individuals shift from being dependent on finding employment in the labour market, to being in receipt of an independent income guaranteed by the taxable capacity of the state. In Edwardian Britain, for example, the average working-class adult had accumulated assets of about £11, at a time when the wage for an unskilled worker was around £1 a week. About 5 per cent of the manual work-force was enrolled in an occupational pension scheme, and well under 5 per cent owned their own property: in consequence, most old people depended on selling their labour power in an over-stocked labour market in order to live.[16] The payment of the state non-contributory old age pension from 1909 gave elderly people a *right* to an income from the state, quite independent of the vicissitudes of the

67

labour market, and this obviously increased their financial independence. Recent arguments about whether the level of state pensions has or has not risen over time relative to average adult per capita income, about whether pensions should or should not be more generous today, and about how criteria for change in the level of pension payments should be set, are all important, but they are essentially distinct from the issue of whether the receipt of state benefits necessarily creates a dependency in the recipient which would not otherwise exist.

One indication of the importance of state pensions in increasing the financial security and independence of the bulk of the British population can be drawn from statistics of wealth distribution in England and Wales collected for the Royal Commission on the Distribution of Income and Wealth. In the early years of this century, before state pensions were introduced, and when occupational pension schemes covered only a small part of the work-force, the bulk of the wealth of the population was held in the form of realizable assets, and was highly concentrated in the hands of a small minority. This has not changed: in 1972, people in the bottom 80 per cent of the wealth distribution owned only 10 per cent of realizable assets. However, realizable assets are now much less important in any estimation of the wealth distribution in Britain, because so much of the wealth of individuals is held in the form of pension rights, wealth which is not immediately realizable, but which is contingent on survival beyond pensionable age. Because private-pension wealth is much more widely spread across the population than are realizable assets, and state-pension wealth is divided among all citizens, the inclusion of these two additional types of assets in a calculation of wealth distribution changes the overall picture drastically. The addition of occupational pension rights to an estimate of the share of wealth owned by the poorest 80 per cent of the popuation in 1972 raises the figure from 10 per cent to 20 per cent, and including state-pension rights doubles this again to over 40 per cent.[17] In other words, the introduction and extension of state-pension rights over the course of the twentieth century has been by far the most important mechanism for increasing the effective wealth of the poorer sections of the population. Without state pensions, many elderly people would be deprived of access to any substantial financial resources in their old age. Although the primary importance of state benefits in financing old age may decline in the future as both the opportunities and the incentives increase for today's working population to accumulate private assets for retirement, there can be little doubt that over the last eighty years state pensions have been instrumental in sustaining a considerable degree of economic independence among the retired population.

Private saving

This financial independence has also been increased by the extension of asset ownership among elderly people. The development of occupational pension schemes, and the rapid increase of owner-occupation since the 1950s, has given many elderly people far more economic security in old age than they ever had when they were reliant on the sale of their labour power. One consequence of the rise in private asset ownership among elderly people is that many of them do not suffer any drastic reduction of their ability to consume on retirement: indeed, tax changes in the 1970s that encouraged pension schemes to pay out some of their assets as a lump sum mean that many retirees experience an increase in their consumption propensity in the first few years of retirement. This may be a powerful influence in any decision about age of retirement. Since the level of owner-occupation is rising, and the number of future retirees entitled to some form of contributory pension will exceed the current number, it seems likely that private saving will play a greater role in determining the economic status of the elderly in the future than it has done in the past. This shift in the economic status of the elderly from being predominantly without assets in the early years of this century towards having at least some private financial resources must represent an overall increase in the economic independence of the elderly population.

Family support

The fourth source of financial support for elderly people is the family, but changes in family support over time are difficult to measure and difficult to interpret. A reduction in the level of intergenerational exchange within the family can be viewed either as an indicator of the increased independence of elderly people, or as a sign of their growing neglect by younger family members. Work by Chris Gordon on elderly people surveyed by the *New Survey of London Life and Labour* in 1929–31 showed that only 7.3 per cent of the 2,286 elderly people in his sample were in receipt of any direct financial support from their family, and this accounted for only 2 per cent of the overall income of this elderly population (as shown in Table 3.1).[18] The household structure of this sample population had many similarities with that observed today: those living alone comprised 29.8 per cent of the elderly population (as against 33.3 per cent in the 1980 GHS),[19] though the proportion living with children or other kin was higher — 34 per cent as against 18 per cent today. It seems likely that the apparent increase in the residential segregation of the elderly since the inter-war period reflects both the substantial rise in the housing stock in recent years (from 16.2

million to 20.5 million units between 1961 and 1981) and the increased financial resources of elderly people, which together have allowed more of them to continue to live private and independent lives.

Table 3.1 Main components of pensioners' income (%)

	Earnings	State benefits	Occup. pension	Savings Investment income	Family
1929–31	35	44	5[a]	14[b]	2
1951	27	42	15	15	—
1961	22	48	16	15	—
1971	18	48	21	10	—
1981–2	10	59	21	10	—
1984–5	9	60	22	9	—

Source: for 1929–31, Chris Gordon, 'Patterns of support for the elderly: the case of London's working class in the early 1930s', MSc dissertation, London School of Economics, 1986. For 1951–85, G.C. Fiegehen, 'Income after retirement', *Social Trends* 16 (1986).
Notes: [a]This includes income from other savings.
[b]This represents income from sub-letting.

Conclusion

Table 3.1 lists the four factors which determine the financial status of elderly people — employment, state benefits, private savings, and family transfers — and it can be seen that their relative shares have changed over time, with the decline in employment income roughly matching the rise in state benefits. It cannot be concluded from this, however, that the economic dependency of the elderly population has increased. Only if it is believed that independence is a function of employment income can the idea of increased dependency be automatically supported. It seems probable that elderly people as a whole have more secure incomes and are less marginalized as consumers today than they were at earlier times in this century.

Of course, considering the financial status of the elderly population as a whole provides only a partial answer to questions which need to be addressed. Within this group there was and remains great variation in financial status by age, class, and gender. Differences in lifetime economic and employment status are carried over into retirement through private asset ownership, and these differences have possibly not diminished significantly. On the other hand, the increase in the importance of state benefits must have tended to reduce the inequality in the economic circumstances of the elderly that hitherto was determined in the labour market.

The idea that old age dependency in twentieth-century Britain has increased, as prepounded in the writing on 'structured dependency', can therefore be seen to be highly contestable. In terms of their asset owner-ship and their household structure, elderly people today have greater command over resources and are less dependent on the goodwill of their kin than was the case in the early years of the twentieth century. In terms of their income, they are less dependent on the vagaries of the labour market, since the major part of their income today is guaranteed by the taxable capacity of the state, and is paid to them as a right. It is certainly true that employment opportunities for older men have declined sharply over the last eighty years, but it is far from clear that this has been solely due to a contraction of demand for them. Improved economic status now gives more elderly people the option of a fairly comfortable retirement which they may prefer to continued employment in unattrac-tive work. What part of any contraction in the demand for elderly workers has been caused by state action over the setting of pension eligibility terms, and what part has been due to the autonomous decisions of employers, must for the moment remain an open question. Indeed, the whole issue of how and why employers (and trade unions) formulate policy towards the employment of older workers requires much more detailed investigation than it has so far received, and it is an area in which economic analysis may prove to be more fruitful than radical political theory.

Notes

1. This chapter is based on research funded by the Economic and Social Research Council (ESRC), reference number GOO 23 2344. It is a shortened version of a longer paper, the full version of which can be obtained from the author on request.
2. Some of the most important works are: Peter Townsend, 'The structured dependency of the elderly: a creation of social policy in the twentieth century', *Ageing and Society* 1 (1981); Chris Phillipson, *Capitalism and the Construc-tion of Old Age* (London, 1982); Alan Walker, 'The social creation of poverty and dependency in old age', *Journal of Social Policy* 9 (1980); 'Towards a political economy of old age', *Ageing and Society* 1 (1981); 'Dependency and old age', *Social Policy and Administration* 16 (1982).
3. Townsend, op. cit., p. 23.
4. Walker, 'Dependency and old age', p. 129.
5. For example, Townsend, op. cit., pp. 13–22; T.A. Booth and others, 'Dependency in residential homes for the elderly', *Social Policy and Administration* 17 (1983): 46–62.
6. Townsend, op. cit., p. 23.
7. Richard Smith, 'The structured dependence of the elderly as a recent develop-ment: some sceptical historical thoughts', *Ageing and Society* 4 (1984); David Thomson, 'The decline of social welfare: falling state support for the elderly since early Victorian times', *Ageing and Society* 4 (1984).

8. David Thomson, 'Welfare and the historians', in L. Bonfield and others (eds) *The World We Have Gained* (Oxford: Basil Blackwell, 1986), pp. 355–78.
9. All these data are drawn from decennial census reports on the occupied population.
10. Phillipson, op. cit., pp. 16–17.
11. Alan Walker, 'Social policy and elderly people in Great Britain', in Anne-Marie Guillemard (ed.) *Old Age and the Welfare State* (London: Sage Publications, 1983), p. 152.
12. Leslie Hannah, *Inventing Retirement* (Cambridge: Cambridge University Press, 1986).
13. Phillipson, op. cit., Chapter 3.
14. Ben Fischer and Edward Montgomery, 'Social security and labour market policy', Chapter 4 of *Fifty Years of Social Security: Past Achievements and Future Challenges*, information paper for the Special Committee on Ageing, US Senate (US Government Printing Office, Washington, DC, August 1985).
15. Walker, 'Dependency and old age', p. 117.
16. Paul Johnson, *Saving and Spending: The Working-class Economy in Britain, 1870–1939* (Oxford: Oxford University Press, 1985), Chapters 3 and 7.
17. The figures are taken from C.D. Harbury and D.M.W.N. Hitchens, *Inheritance and Wealth Inequality in Britain* (London: Allen and Unwin, 1979), and are derived from the Royal Commission on the Distribution of Income and Wealth, Report No. 1, 1975 (Cmnd. 6171).
18. Chris Gordon, 'Patterns of support for the elderly: the case of London's working class in the early 1930s', MSc Dissertation, London School of Economics, 1986.
19. *General Household Survey, 1980*, OPCS Social Survey Division (HMSO, London, 1982).

Chapter four

The Social Division of
Early Retirement[1]

Alan Walker

Introduction

Some findings are presented from a recent study of older workers and
early retirement in the Sheffield steel industry (under the ESRC Ageing
Initiative). The study consisted of an analysis of data on retirement and
early retirement from the 'After Redundancy' project conducted by Iain
Noble, John Westergaard, and Alan Walker and funded by the Economic
and Social Research Council (ESRC). The results reported are intended
as a contribution to the debate about early retirement as a mechanism
for sharing the current job shortage. They provide a new dimension to
this debate because they derive from the experience of a different socio-
economic group and markedly changed labour market conditions to most
of the previous research on this issue.

The after redundancy study

The study was based on structured interviews with some 370 former
employees of a privately owned steel company in Sheffield who were
made redundant in and shortly after the summer of 1979. The firm's
management approached us in the summer of 1980, asking if we could
find out 'what had happened' to their former employees, and agreed to
provide the names and addresses of those who had lost their jobs. Interviews were conducted between October 1982 and February 1983. The
final response rate was 79 per cent. (A full report of the project's findings
can be found in Westergaard et al 1988.)

Until the early 1980s, unemployment in Sheffield had been below
the national average for the whole of the post-war period. The relative
prosperity of Sheffield was based partly on the production of special steels
(carbon steel, alloy steel, and stainless steel) and related manufacturing
industry. As a result of the cut-back in production by the steel industry's
customers and the 'dumping' of subsidized special steel imports, the
numbers of people employed in metal manufacture have declined

73

enormously in recent years: between mid-1979 and mid-1983 the reduction in the numbers employed in this sector was greater than in any other
sector of the economy (Department of Employment 1983: 511). Thus,
from the late 1970s parts of Sheffield began, very rapidly, to experience
that deterioration of the economic fabric that has been felt in other parts
of the county of South Yorkshire for much longer (Walker 1981).

The majority (55 per cent) of those made redundant by the private
steel firm were older workers (those 55 and over when interviewed).[2]
The analysis reported here was focused on this group. An age bias of
this order was expected — only one in seven were under the age of 30
— because of the relatively high median age of the work-force in the
steel industry (Jolly *et al.* 1980: 91), the greater likelihood of their older
workers than younger ones being affected by redundancies (Mukherjee
1973; Daniel 1974), and the semi-voluntary nature of the redundancies
in question. The gender distribution also followed a predictable pattern,
with the overwhelming majority, 85 per cent, being male. Among the
older age-groups the proportion was even higher: just under 90 per cent.
Thus, it is not possible to say much about the post-redundancy experience
of older women previously employed in this sector of industry. In view
of the relative neglect of women in studies of redundancy, this was an
unfortunate deficiency (see Daniel 1972; Barron and Norris 1978).
However, two further characteristics made this group a particularly
interesting one for the study of the labour market experiences of older
male workers in a period of high unemployment and rapid economic
and social change.

First, two-thirds of them were manual workers. This contrasts with
other recent non-representative research on early retirement, carried out
by McGoldrick and Cooper (1980), which concentrated on those in higher
socio-economic groups (see also S. Wood 1980). They found that the
majority were satisfied with early retirement. Although doubt has been
cast on that finding by the results of the national survey (see Parker 1982:
90), McGoldrick and Cooper's research was conducted after the national
survey and it has helped to encourage a view that attitudes towards early
retirement are changing significantly and that it is being regarded more
and more favourably by older workers (see for example, House of
Commons Select Committee on Social Services 1982). It was important, therefore, to compare the conclusion of that research with the results
of the After Redundancy study which was based on contrasting socio-
economic groups. Moreover, there has been little recent research on what
befalls older manual workers following redundancy, although the labour
market has undergone a period of rapid change over the last few years
(one recent exception is Bytheway 1987).

Second, a large proportion of the older workers had a long period
of service with the same company before being made redundant. Only

17 per cent of the older workers had been with the company for less than ten years (only 5 per cent for less than five years), while 68 per cent had twenty years or more service. More than two-fifths of them had worked in the company for at least thirty years. The majority had therefore experienced secure employment for relatively long periods of time. Thus, we are able to assess the impact of redundancy and unemployment on a group for whom these were rare if not entirely new occurrences. One in six of the older workers had experienced redundancy prior to 1979, over half of them among those with less than ten years service with the company. Again this contrasts with other research which has examined the labour market status of older workers, but which has sampled directly or indirectly among the unemployed (Hill *et al.* 1973; Daniel 1974; D. Wood 1982). Although more representative of the whole unemployed population than the After Redundancy study, research on unemployment alone is insufficient to judge the specific impact of redundancy, especially on older workers — many of whom do not choose to declare themselves as unemployed, so register only while entitled to unemployment benefit — and the experience of economic insecurity following relatively secure employment.

One further contextual factor had an important bearing on this analysis. The After Redundancy study took place during a period when the level of economic activity among older people in general, and older men in particular, had been declining (Walker 1980; Parker 1982; OPCS 1987). Older people in the study had to enter the labour market at precisely the time of the steepest fall in the economic activity rates of older workers at large. The national growth in economic inactivity is also reflected in the increasing trend towards early retirement among some groups of people in the 60–64 age range. Britain shares this changing pattern of retirement with other advanced industrial societies, although there has been no formal lowering of the age at which the statutory retirement-pension may be drawn. (Tracy 1979; OECD 1986).

The impact of redundancy on the employment status of older workers

Older workers (aged 55 and over) in the After Redundancy study were less likely than older workers as a whole to be economically active. By the time they were interviewed in late 1982 and early 1983 (some three years after being made redundant), they were divided almost equally between the economically active and inactive — 51 per cent and 49 per cent respectively — according to the standard definition of such activity.[3] However, in common with some previous research (Sinfield 1968; Norris 1978; Townsend 1979; Walker 1982a), the results of the After Redundancy study raised questions about the precise distinctions between economic activity and inactivity and especially about the assumptions which underlie this crude dichotomy, a point I return to later.

Among those older workers in the study conventionally defined as economically inactive, just over two-thirds were retired, although only 18 per cent had retired at the normal pension age, 17 per cent were sick or injured, and 4 per cent were looking after their families. As for the economically active, 56 per cent were employed full- or part-time and 44 per cent were unemployed. Before they became redundant some three years earlier, all of them had been economically active and in full-time employment.

Figure 4.1 shows the employment status of two age-groups of older workers immediately after redundancy and three years later at the time of interview. The impact of redundancy on the employment status of older workers was remarkable, with only one in six of all those aged 55 and over moving from employment with the steel company to a further spell of employment, and only one in seven to full-time work. Although these proportions changed subsequently, particularly among the 55–59 age group, after three years only one in four of the whole group (excluding those who had retired at the normal pension ages) were in work. In contrast three-quarters of those under 40 at the time of interview and three-fifths of the middle-aged (40–54) were employed after three years. Nearly all of the former and two in three of the latter went straight into jobs after they were made redundant. Figure 4.1 shows the distribution of employment statuses at two points in time. If all the positions occupied in the intervening three years were included, the picture would, of course, be a great deal more complicated.

The figure also shows that there were important differences in post-redundancy employment status among older workers based on age, or rather, on their proximity to state-pension age. Initially the flow out of the labour force and into retirement was concentrated among men within three years of pension age. Three years after redundancy the picture had changed, with the level of employment rising among those still under pension age and the level of unemployment falling. However, whereas for the 55–59 age-group the fall in unemployment was compensated for by an increase in employment, as well as in sickness and disability, for the 60–64 age-group early retirement increased more substantially than employment. The pattern of changes in status over the three years since redundancy was broadly similar for those aged 55–59, 40–54, and under 40 at the time of redundancy. However, for those aged 60–64 the pattern is quite different, the clear difference in the direction of the flows is indicated by the arrows in the Figure 4.1. (For a detailed account of the post-redundancy experiences of all of the older workers in the study see Walker *et al.* 1985).

With cross-sectional data it is not possible to make precise comparisons between changes in employment and economic activity over time.

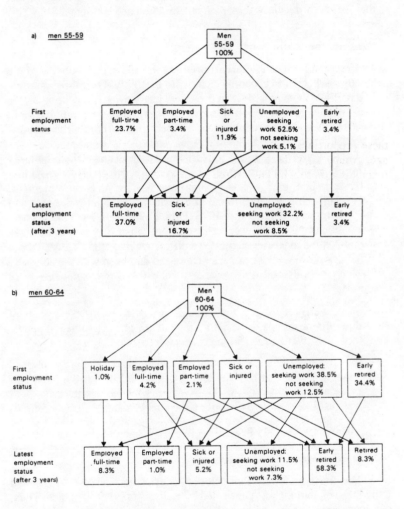

Figure 4.1 Employment status of older male workers following redundancy according to age at time of redundancy

However, we collected detailed information on the employment and labour market histories of respondents in the three years between redundancy and interview, and previous research indicates that such information can be collected reliably for such relatively short periods (Walker 1982a). The following analysis uses these post-redundancy histories as a guide to some of the influences on older workers when they came to decide whether or not to take early retirement.

Reasons for taking early retirement

As Figure 4.1 indicates, early retirement was the major route out of the labour market, from economic activity to inactivity. Over three-quarters of those who were retired when they were interviewed had done so before pension age. Just over half of those who retired prematurely did so at the same time as their redundancy. The rest took early retirement at different points over the following three years.

There were four main characteristics which distinguished the early retired from other older people. First, age, or more precisely proximity to the state-pension age, had an important bearing on early retirement. This relationship was also found in the national study of retirement and early retirement, conducted in 1977 (Parker 1980: 13). Answers to questions about their fellow workers' reactions when they heard the news of planned redundancies suggested a difference in attitude between some of those who were close to pension age and had been with the company for long periods and other workers. The following comments were typical:

> Some were very angry, they thought it would last for ever; yes a bit down in the dumps, especially the younger people, some old people looked forward to it. (Man 65, early retired)

> It just depends, some of them were laughing, they were pleased enough. Those that had any length of time in, they had a hand-out. Quite a few were very upset, they'd only twelve months to go — it was just like turning them out on the street. (Man, 66, early retired)

> The older ones were pleased because they would get a lot of money, the younger ones were upset because they were thinking about the future. (Man, 58, early retired)

The division between those close to pension age and others suggested by these quotations was confirmed by analysis of other variables. Thus, for example, when asked whether or not they would describe their own redundancy as genuinely voluntary, the oldest group (those over 65 when interviewed) were much more likely than the rest to say 'yes' (83 per cent compared with 46 per cent of those aged 55–59 and 65 per cent of those aged 60–64). Furthermore, they were less likely to have applied to be taken on by the firm's main competitor, which took over its order book, or to look for another job before leaving the firm.

Because a detailed record of economic activity statuses was collected by the After Redundancy study, it was possible to compare the proportion of time spent by each person since being made redundant in different forms of employment status. When older workers were compared on the basis of their proximity to pension age when the redundancies took place, the proportion of the three years between redundancy and interview spent in retirement increased dramatically, the closer they were to pension age. Thus, the mean proportion of time spent retired by those within 4–6 years of pension age was 19 per cent, compared with 57 per cent of those within 3–4 years, and 84 per cent of those with 1–2 years to go before reaching pension age.

Second, we found that ill health was an important factor in the decision to retire early, although it was not possible to say whether or not it was the overriding factor. Certainly, when asked directly why they had decided to take early retirement, it was the most frequently mentioned reason by those concerned. This finding corresponds with research that has concentrated on early retirement (McGoldrick and Cooper 1980; Parker 1980; and in France, Cribier 1981; Gaullier 1982) and withdrawal from the labour market through the job release scheme (Makeham and Morgan 1980: 14), but we do not know how many of those older workers with poor health would have been fit enough to continue working if the plant had not closed. Some had been finding work a strain and early retirement came as a relief. Others were sick and disabled, yet still wanted paid employment (see Figure 4.1). In fact, the dividing lines were often difficult to draw between those formally described as sick and those described as early-retired. It appears that severity of illness or disability is likely to have been a critical variable, and in cases of severe disability, health would have been an overriding consideration. More commonly, however, it was ill health in conjunction with other factors, such as proximity to retirement age, which determined propensity to retire early. Ironically, there were some respondents who said that they would have preferred to have kept on working in order to remain healthy. In the words of one 66 year-old man, 'It keeps you fit and healthy, gives you something to occupy your mind, and you don't get bored.'

Third, our study confirmed the finding of previous research (Friedmann and Orbach 1974; McGoldrick and Cooper 1980; Parker 1980) that the individual's own or his or her income unit's financial resources had an important bearing on the decision to retire early. Although those older workers in full-time employment were substantially better off than other groups, the early retired were better off than the rest. They were more than three times as likely as the unemployed to be part of an income unit with an income of more than £100 per week (14 per cent and 4 per cent) and half as likely to have an income of less than £50 a week (19 per cent and 41 per cent).

Of course the redundancy payment was an important source of capital for many older workers and, therefore, contributed to the decision about early retirement. More than two-thirds of those aged 60 or over when interviewed had received a redundancy payment of £3,000 or more. Those with the longer periods received higher payments than those with shorter periods and were more likely to have retired early. This was another way in which redundancy encouraged some older workers to take early retirement. Some older workers feared that if they did not accept 'voluntary' redundancy they would not receive any redundancy pay. When early retirement took place at the same time as redundancy, the fear of not getting financial compensation became a reason for taking early retirement.

Fourth, differences in financial status between the early retired and other workers were underpinned by social class (based on occupational group). Thus, there was a clear distinction in the social-class distribution of early retirement between the semi-skilled and unskilled, who were most likely to wait until the statutory pension ages (64 per cent of those retired had retired early), and the supervisory and managerial group, most of whom (95 per cent) had retired early. The proportion of retired skilled workers who did so prematurely fell between these two at 79 per cent.

The importance of social class membership in providing access to resources, including income, was demonstrated by the fact that differences betweem the propensity of those in different classes to retire early increased with distance from pension age. Taking those within 1–2 years of the pension age first, non-manual workers had spent nearly one-third more of the intervening time between redundancy and interview in retirement than skilled manual workers (85.7 per cent and 66.8 per cent respectively). For those within 2–4 years of the pension age, the comparative figures were 76.7 per cent and 59.3 per cent and for those with 4–6 years before pension age, 37.9 per cent compared with 7.7 per cent. The differences suggest that those in the non-manual occupational groups were more likely to choose early retirement than skilled manual workers, presumably because thay had greater resources and hence more freedom of choice.

Pressure on older workers to take early retirement

These then are the main characteristics which distinguish the early retired from other older workers who remained actually or potentially in the labour market: the former were more likely to have been close to pension age, to report ill health, to be better off financially and to have non-manual occupations. On their own, however, these supply-side characteristics do not explain fully why a significant proportion of older workers were early-retired. In order to do so it is necessary also to consider demand-side factors.

Frequently, early retirement is discussed purely in individualistic terms — as if it were a matter simply of personal decision-making. In some cases, certainly, it is the result of a free choice on the part of individuals, most of whom are concentrated in the higher social classes where financial security, other than through earned income, is common. Research which has suggested that there has been an increase in voluntary early retirement has been based on the responses of financially secure early retirees (see, for example, Heidbreder 1972; McGoldrick and Cooper 1980). More representative research, such as that conducted by Parker (1980) in this country and Schwab (1976) and her colleagues in the USA, found that voluntary early retirement was relatively rare. However, even research which has concentrated on the decision to take voluntary early retirement by those who have been able to exercise choice relatively freely, while still in employment, has noted external pressures on the individuals concerned (see, for example, McGoldrick and Cooper 1980: 860).

The social-class differences in early retirement revealed by our study point to clear divisions in the degree of choice available to individuals. Ill health, for example, may be as much a demand-side as a supply-side factor through social pressures on those who suffer it to take early retirement at a time of general contraction. In addition, there is the most important demand-side pressure — namely, changes in the demand for labour locally and nationally, the effects of which have been largely overlooked in previous research.

First, there is redundancy itself, which was undoubtedly the main spur to early retirement among those in the After Redundancy study. If the steel plant had not closed down, most of the early-retired would have probably stayed in their jobs until the pension age. Although it is impossible to be certain, this assumption is supported by the overall length of service of the majority, their attachment to the particular employer, as well as their answers to specific questions about redundancy and early retirement. Thus, for example, when asked whether they had ever thought seriously about early retirement before the prospect of redundancy was raised, less than one-quarter had done so. In fact, those who retired prematurely were less likely than those who waited until pension age to have said that they had ever thought seriously about early retirement (24 per cent compared with 44 per cent in the age-group 60 and over).

If the plant had not closed, there would undoubtedly have been some older workers who would have retired prematurely in any case. However, for the majority of those that eventually retired early, redundancy appears to have been the deciding factor. This is true even where respondents reported ill health or dissatisfacton with work.

Our study did not find any evidence of widespread dissatisfaction among older workers with either their employment or their employer prior to plant closure. Indeed, they were much more likely than their younger counterparts to have expressed satisfaction with the firm and its management. Thus, older workers were more than twice as likely as those under 40 to say that they had a great deal of respect for the top management at the firm (72 per cent). However, although only one in twenty of those over the age of 55 reported that they were pleased about the plant closure, those who did so were concentrated almost entirely in the group that was within three years of pension age when the redundancies took place. Proximity to pension age therefore had a significant impact on attitudes towards redundancy and the end of working life it signalled.

Secondly, there is the level of demand for labour locally, and, particularly, the demand for older workers with specific skills. High and rising unemployment in Sheffield and knowledge about the poor employment prospects of older workers already in the labour market contributed to the decisions made about early retirement in two ways. On the one hand, the local situation and knowledge about it encouraged some people to retire at the same time as they were made redundant. As soon as the redundancies were announced, just over half of those who retired before the pension age decided that they did not want to go through the process of trying to find work. They did so in the face of widespread steel closures, rising unemployment, and knowledge about their poor prospects of re-employment, or they had had enough of work and felt they deserved a rest.

On the other hand, there was a slightly smaller group of people, ending up as early retired, who had at first decided to remain economically active and, for the most part, to try to find jobs. This group was likely to be younger than the first. Although a minority of the group succeeded in finding jobs, these did not last long, and, like the rest of this group, who remained unemployed, they became frustrated and disillusioned by the difficulties they experienced in finding employment and by the attitude of employers to older workers. As a result, they decided to change their economic status from either unemployment or sickness to early retirement. In early retirement older workers have a socially acceptable alternative to the stigma of unemployment, that is not available to younger people (Bruche and Casey 1982: 112); but first they must get close to pension age.

One critical aspect of the overall decline in the demand for labour was the discrimination that older workers believed employers exercised against them and in favour of younger ones. Objective evidence of employers' bias in the recruitment was found by Jolly *et al.* (1980). Nearly all the unemployed men aged 60–64 in our study mentioned the bias towards younger people in recruitment. Not surprisingly, job applications tended to be concentrated in the early stages of unemployment and to cease when older workers became discouraged from making further, fruitless efforts.

Thirdly, official labour market intermediaries in the job centres are an important source of information about employment prospects and a crucial part of the process of discouraging older workers from searching for work and, indirectly, of encouraging them to take early retirement. For many older people in our study the process began as soon as they were registered as unemployed. They were much less likely than younger people to be interviewed by job centre staff, and, if interviewed, they were more likely to be told their prospects of getting work were nil.

Finally, there is the economic and social policy context within which older workers come to a decision about whether or not to remain economically active. Attitudes towards employment, retirement, and early retirement are not formed in a vacuum. In addition to the long-term devaluation of the industrial worth of older people (Walker 1980; Phillipson 1982), the last eight years, including the periods leading up to and immediately after the redundancies under study took place, were marked by frequent references to the need for earlier retirement. These were accompanied, more importantly, by social policies aimed at encouraging early retirement.

As unemployment began to rise rapidly in the late 1970s, early retirement was canvassed, more and more and by an increasingly diverse range of opinion, as a solution to the problem. The Confederation of British Industry and Trades Union Congress have both given their support to a reduction in the male pension age, as have the House of Lords Select Committee on Unemployment (1982) and the House of Commons Select Committee on Social Services (1982). The Labour Party's manifestos at the last two general elections contained proposals to lower the main retirement age. At the same time, official and mass media attention has been concentrated on youth unemployment and the problems experienced by young people in the labour market. Employment policy too has been directed overwhelmingly towards this group.

In contrast, the few policies aimed at older workers have been positively intended to encourage them to withdraw from the labour market. Measures have been introduced recently in the spheres of employment and social security. The most important policy in the field of employment is the Job Release Scheme, introduced in 1977 as a temporary measure for men aged 64 and women aged 59 and extended in 1981 and 1982 to cover disabled men aged 60–63 and other men aged 62 and 63. It is intended to 'alleviate unemployment among younger workers' (DHSS 1981: 16) by replacing older workers with them. Those taking up job-release allowances must not take a job or set up in business on their own, and their employer must undertake to recruit as soon as possible a registered unemployed worker. The number taking part was expected to exceed 100,000.

In social security there is the retirement condition, which governs the receipt of the state retirement pension and which has been a major factor in the establishment of the pension ages as the customary retirement ages for men and women (Walker 1980). Similarly, the introduction of age- and service-related redundancy payments in 1965 to some extent legitimated the use of age as a criterion for redundancy and successfully challenged the 'first in last out' principle (Mukherjee 1973: 107). Between November 1981 and November 1983, encouragement was given to unemployed men over the age of 60 to withdraw from the labour force by offering to pay them the long-term rate of supplementary benefit if they agreed not to register as unemployed. Although this change in policy meant that unemployed older workers could receive a one-fifth increase in their weekly benefit income, the majority in our study had chosen to retire early *before* November 1981. In other words, there was no clear evidence that the level of social security benefits was a major factor in the early retirement decisions made by those in this study (Boskin 1977: Burkhauser and Tolley 1978; Haveman and Wolfe 1981).

Together, these policies and policy statements reflect an overwhelming official concern in the current period of high unemployment with the position of young people in the labour market and, conversely, a lack of interest in action to improve the employment prospects of older workers. They reflect, in other words, an increasing tendency, directly or indirectly, to discriminate against older people in favour of younger ones, or 'ageism' (Walker 1982b). In turn, this strong bias affects the climate of opinion in society as a whole, but especially in the labour market, where it influences employers. personnel officers, job centre staff, and other officials and, of course, older workers themselves. In December 1982 a Marplan public opinion poll found that four out of five of those questioned thought that early retirement was a desirable measure for alleviating unemployment. In the After Redundancy study, support for compulsory retirement at an earlier age was nearly as widespread, with one-third saying it would be very effective and two-fifths saying it would be quite effective. Moreover, it was those that were most likely to suffer long periods of unemployment and non-employment and for whom early retirement was a realistic option, i.e. those aged 60–64, who were most likely to say that it would be very effective in dealing with unemployment: 46 per cent, compared wth 34 per cent of the 55–59 age-group and 30 per cent of those under 30.

Statements by individuals in response to questions about early retirement also often reflected the dominant official concern. Not surprisingly, older workers themselves had apparently internalized the assumptions which underpin policy, including the priority to be given to young people. The terms respondents used to describe the advantages of early retirement, or to rationalize it in retrospect, often showed concern for the position of young people in the labour market, although this was rarely cited as a reason for taking early retirement. One man who took early retirement at 61 thought, at the time, that the advantage of early retirement was 'The fact that there are so many young people out of work and I thought I'd done a lifetime's work and might as well leave it for the young ones.' Similar comments were reported by McGoldrick and Cooper (1980: 860).

Thus, the policy context, within which the redundancies took place and which older workers experienced in the labour market, often for the first time in twenty or more years, was one of unconcern if not of antagonism to their special needs. Official and public attitudes towards older workers — which to a large extent determine the extent of their inclusion in or exclusion from the labour force — rest primarily on the damand for labour. Thus, in contrast with current policies, in the period immediately after the Second World War people of retirement age were urged *not* to retire and to 'sink into premature old age', but to work a little longer and, therefore, have 'a happier and healthier old age' (Phillipson 1982: 33). At the same time, medical and social science research began to indicate that retirement itself had detrimental effects.

Today, a formal lowering of the male retirement age to 60 has been rejected on grounds of cost, but high rates of unemployment among the 60–64 age-group, together with official encouragement for unemployed men to leave the labour force, amounts to an informal *de facto* policy of increasing early retirement for men. While such a policy may relieve the short-term burden of unemployment for the older men nearest retirement age, unfortunately our study showed that the majority of those in their mid- and late fifties, who did not have the option of becoming early retired, faced the prospect of very long-term unemployment, and found the experience very distressing (Walker *et al.* 1985). Moreover, the possible long-term consequences of current policies, such as deeper poverty in advanced old age, have not yet been sufficiently considered publicly (Walker 1982b: 66–9).

Social exclusion, discouragement, and early retirement

Which of these demand- and supply-related factors exerted a dominant influence on individual older workers in deciding whether or not to cease economic activity and become early retired? The After Redundancy study suggests that it was those on the demand side and, in the first instance, the redundancy itself. When presented with the alternative of long-term unemployment, with no prospect of a job, some semi-skilled and unskilled older workers had no effective choice about early retirement. However, if demand-related factors were dominant, they were not overriding. There were still those in the skilled, supervisory, and managerial groups, who might have sought alternative employment and stood a better chance than the majority of finding it, who chose instead to take early retirement. In these cases, financial security, a reluctance to move to a new employer, and proximity to the statutory pension age, coupled with a desire to do other things with their time or simply to stop working, led them to opt for early retirement. There were also others who felt that they had to stop work because of their own or their spouse's ill health.

For the vast majority of older workers in the After Redundancy study, therefore, it was likely to be the interaction of the two sets of influences — individual characteristics and knowledge about the demand for labour and their chances of securing further employment of a similar kind — that determined their response to redundancy. However, in the absence of financial security, the option of early retirement rested primarily on proximity to pension age (see Figure 4.1).

All those who retired prematurely were forced by redundancy to make a decision about their future employment status. Half of those who retired at that point or subsequently were effectively forced into early retirement by ill health or the lack of job opportunities. Only three of the whole group had worked since redundancy, and only one of those did so for more than half of the time between redundancy and interview. As a result, for the bulk of those who delayed a decision about early retirement, unemployment or sickness amounted to a similar economic status to early retirement: non-employment. However, considerably more social stigma is attached to unemployment than to early retirement. In addition, for those men aged 60–64 after November 1981, a simple change in the official label attached to their status would have resulted in an increase in their income by one-fifth. Thus, the formal decision to retire prematurely, when it came, was not simply a rationalization of the individual's situation, but a considerable improvement in it both economically and socially.

In sum, two approaches to early retirement may be distinguished. On the one hand, there were those who, once the prospect of redundancy had been raised, were reconciled to early retirement and to a greater or lesser extent relieved at leaving work, although they were attached to their employer and would not in all probability have left prematurely of their own volition. On the other hand, there were those who gave up work reluctantly and would have preferred to have kept on working, but for reasons of health or lack of alternative employment chose early retirement.

The early retirers in the After Redundancy study were split evenly between those who wanted to retire and those who would have preferred to work on. (This compares, incidentally, with just over one-quarter of those who retired at the normal pension ages who would have preferred to keep on working.) With the exception of a few of the non-manual workers, concentrated in the first group, early retirement cannot be said to have been chosen from a position of strength — namely, possessing financial security, good health, and the option of continued employment. It was an alternative to secure employment for some who fit the popular image of the early retired, but for others it was a refuge from economic insecurity in the labour market.

Those in the latter group — the reluctant early retirers — conform directly to what have been described in the USA as 'discouraged workers' (Sorrentino 1981: 168; and for a discussion of the discouraged worker effect based on British Labour Force survey data, see Laczko 1987). They are people who would like to work but believe no work is available, lack the schooling, training, skills, or experience required by employers, are thought by employers to be too young or too old or who have other personal handicaps in finding a job. The small number of older (and younger) women who gave up paid employment following redundancy to become housewives may also be included in this group of discouraged workers.

The discouraging effects of prolonged unemployment, experience in the labour market with employers and official intermediaries, public statements by political and economic commentators, politicians, and employers about the future of employment are all part of a social process of exclusion, which probably began to set the agenda in the minds of individual older workers in the After Redundancy study even before the redundancy itself took place.

The process of exclusion in operation currently is an important part of the social construction of the definition and redefinition of the labour force, of the economically active and inactive, of the unemployed and retired, of the productive and unproductive, and, therefore, of working age and old age (Walker 1980; Phillipson, 1982). It is the process whereby the state encourages and legitimates certain forms of dependency, such as unemployment and early retirement among men aged 60–64, while subjecting others not only to substantially lower incomes, but also to control procedures intended to ensure that they continue searching for work (Sinfield 1981: 142).

Conclusion

Large-scale early retirement is a relatively new phenomenon in Britain. It has become an important aspect of the response by both government and individual older workers to the current continuing economic recession in the labour market. Yet surprisingly little research has been conducted into the subject, at least in Britain. The results of the special analysis of the After Redundancy study reported here add to previous research by showing that early retirement must be seen, not only as an alternative to secure employment, but as economic insecurity as well. Furthermore, they emphasise the point that, like redundancy (Lee and Harris 1985), early retirement must be considered as a *process* rather than an event. This process includes demand factors, such as the demand for labour and employer discrimination, as well as redundancy itself, which may precipitate early retirement; and supply factors, such as the incomes and health of older workers. Policy has developed on the basis not only of inadequate knowledge about the factors contributing to early retirement, but also without any information about the longer-term consequences for the older people involved.

The study was not concerned mainly with early retirement, and the information it did collect was directed primarily towards early retirement as a response to redundancy. Further research is required if we are to understand better the process of early retirement in a variety of circumstances and thereby build a sounder basis for policy. The longer experience of some other countries, such as France and Sweden, of both early retirement and labour market policies encouraging it, would be one potentially fruitful source of information (Walker and Laczko 1982: Laczko and Walker 1985). This study has helped to pave the way for further work on early retirement by showing that, even among the same cohort of redundant workers, there is a clear social division based on economic security and insecurity. Early retirement may be a release from employment for some and a refuge from the severe insecurity of the labour market for others.

Notes

1. This chapter is an abbreviated form of a revised version of a paper published in *The Quarterly Journal of Social Affairs* 1(3) (1985). The full revised version can be obtained from the author on request.
2. Unless otherwise stated the age used throughout this report is age at the time of interview (i.e. three years after redundancy).
3. 'Economically active' includes those in employment and unemployed. 'Economically inactive' includes the retired, housewives, those aged 16 and over in full-time education, thsoe aged under 16, and the permanently sick and disabled (see OPCS 1982: 14).

References

Barron, R.D. and Norris, G.M. (1978) 'Sexual divisions in the dual labour market', in D. Barker and S. Allen (eds) *Dependence and Exploitation in Work and Marriage*, London: Longman, pp. 47–69.

Boskin, M.J. (1977) 'Social security and retirement decisions', *Economic Inquiry* XV: 1–25.

Bruche, G. and Casey, B. (1982) *Work or Retirement*, Berlin: International Institute of Management.

Burkhauser, R.V. and Tolley, G.S. (1978) 'Older Americans and market work', *The Gerontologist* 18 (5): 449–53.

Bytheway, B. (1987) 'Redundancy and the Older Worker', in R. Lee (ed.) *Redundancy Lay Offs and Plant Closures*, Beckenham: Croom Helm, pp. 84–115.

Cribier, F. (1981) 'Changing retirement patterns of the seventies: the examples of a generation of Parisian salaried workers', *Ageing and Society* 1(1): 51–72.

Daniel, W.W. (1972) *Whatever Happened to the Workers in Woolwich?*, London: PEP.

Daniel, W.W. (1974) *National Survey of the Unemployed*, London: PEP.

Department of Employment (1983) *Employment Gazette* 91(11), November.

DHSS (1981) *Growing Older*, Cmnd. 8173, London: HMSO.

Friedmann, E.A. and Orbach, H.L. (1974) 'Adjustment to Retirement', in S. Arieti (ed.) *American Handbook of Psychiatry*, vol. 1 New York: Basic Books.

Gaullier, X. (1982) 'Economic Crisis and Old Age: Old Age Policies in France', *Ageing and Society*, 2(2), pp. 165–82.

Haveman, R.H. and Wolfe, B.L. (1981) 'Have disability transfers caused the decline in older male labour force participation?', University of Wisconsin-Madison, Institute for Research on Poverty.

Heidbreder, E.M. (1972) 'Factors in retirement adjustment: white collar/blue collar experience', *Industrial Gerontology* 12: 69–79.

Hill, M.J., Harrison, R.M., Sargeant, A.V., and Talbot, V. (1973) *Men Out of Work*, Cambridge: Cambridge University Press.

House of Commons Select Committee on Social Services (1982) *Age of Retirement*, HC 26, London: HMSO.

House of Lords Select Committee on Unemployment (1982) *Volume 1 — Report*, HL 142, London: HMSO.

Jolly, J., Creigh, S., and Mingay, A. (1980) *Age as a Factor in Employment*, London: Department of Employment.

Laczko, F. (1987) 'Older workers, unemployment, and the discouraged worker effect', in S. Di Gregorio (ed.) *Social Gerontology: New Directions*, Beckenham: Croom Helm, pp. 239–51.

Laczko, F., and Walker, A. (1985) 'Excluding older workers from the labour market: early retirement in Britain, France and Sweden', in C. Jones and M. Brenton (eds) *The Year Book of Social Policy in Britain*, London: Routledge & Kegan Paul.

Lee, R.M. and Harris, C.C. (1985) 'Redundancy studies: Port Talbot and the future', *Quarterly Journal of Social Affairs* 1(1): 19–27.

McGoldrick, A. and Cooper, C. (1980) 'Voluntary early retirement — Taking the decision', *Employment Gazette*, August: 859–64.

Makeham, P. and Morgan, P. (1980) *Evaluation of the Job Release Scheme*, London: Department of Employment.

Mukherjee, S. (1973) *Through No Fault of Their Own*, London: Macdonald/PEP.

Norris, G. (1978) 'Unemployment, subemployment and personal characteristics', *Sociological Review* 26: 89–103.

OECD (1986) *Early Retirement Policies*, Paris: OECD.

OPCS (1982) *Labour Force Survey 1979*, London: HMSO.

OPCS (1987) *General Household Survey 1986*, London: HMSO.

Parker, S. (1980) *Older Workers and Retirement*, London: HMSO.

Parker, S. (1982) *Work and Retirement*, London: George Allen & Unwin.

Phillipson, C. (1982) *Capitalism and the Construction of Old Age*, London: Macmillan.

Schwab, K. (1976) 'Early labour-force withdrawal of men: participants and non-participants aged 58–63'. in L.M. Irelan *et al. Almost 65: Baseline Data from the Retirement History Study*, Washington, DC: DHEW, pp. 43–56.

Showler, B. and Sinfield, A. (eds) (1981) *The Workless State*, Oxford: Martin Robertson.

Sinfield, A. (1968) *The Long-term Unemployed*, Paris: OECD.

Sinfield, A. (1981) 'Unemployment in an unequal society', in Showler and Sinfield (eds), pp. 122–6.

Sorrentino, C. (1981) 'Unemployment in international perspective', in Showler and Sinfield (eds), pp. 167–214.

Townsend, P. (1979) *Poverty in the United Kingdom*, Harmondsworth: Penguin.

Tracy, M. (1979) *Retirement Age Practices in Ten Industrial Societies, 1960–1976*, Geneva: ISSA.

Walker, A. (1980) 'The social creation of poverty and dependency in old age', *Journal of Social Policy* 9(1): 49–75.

Walker, A. (1981) 'South Yorkshire: the economic and social impact of unemployment', in B. Crick (ed.) *Unemployment*, London: Methuen, pp. 74–87.

Walker, A. (1982a) Unqualified and Underemployed, London: Macmillan.

Walker, A. (1982b) 'The social consequences of early retirement', *Political Quarterly* 53(1): 61–72.

Walker, A. and Laczko, F. (1982) 'Early retirement and flexible retirement', in Social Services Committee, *Age of Retirement*, HC 26–II, London: HMSO, pp. 211–29.

Walker, A., Noble, I., and Westergaard, J. (1985) 'From secure employment to labour market insecurity', in R. Finnegan, D. Gallie, and B. Roberts (eds) *New Aproaches to Economic Life*, Manchester: Manchester University Press.

Westergaard, J., Noble, I. and Walker, A. (1988) *After Redundancy: The Experience of Economic Insecurity*, Oxford, Polity Press.

Wood, D. (1982) *The DHSS Cohort Study of Unemployed Men*, London: DHSS.

Wood, S. (1980) 'Managerial reactions to job redundancy through early retirement', *Sociological Review* 28(4): 783–807.

Part II

Resources in Old Age: Mining National Statistical Sources

Chapter five

Resources in Old Age: Ageing and the Life Course[†]

G. Nigel Gilbert, Angela Dale, Sara Arber, Maria Evandrou, Frank Laczko

Introduction

A number of recent reports have emphasized that 'the elderly' are far from a homogeneous group. Taylor and Ford (1983), for example, examined age, sex, and social-class differences in a sample of elderly people in Aberdeen, finding substantial inequalities between subgroups in their income, social support, health, and psychological functioning. Victor and Evandrou (1986) studied social-class differences using a nationally representative sample from the General Household Survey (GHS) and concluded that the income and health of old people are strongly related to their past employment experience. This chapter explores the relationship between age and several measures of inequality, drawing for our data on a nationally representative sample of elderly people from the GHS. We focus on the significance of 'stage' in life course in accounting for inequality amongst the elderly, and use the analysis to reflect on the likely consequences of current pension and health policies.

Taylor and Ford (1983: 183) note that 'the distinction between the "young" and the "old" elderly is now commonplace' and suggest that this is manifested in, among other factors, the greater likelihood that the old elderly live in poor housing and that they have incomes below or near the supplementary-benefit rate. In the report of the Royal Commission on the Distribution of Incomes (Layard *et al.* 1978), it was shown that, in 1976, the proportion of elderly heads of household with net incomes at or below the supplementary-benefit rate increased from 25 per cent at age 65–69 to 47 per cent at age 80 and over.

Several quite different kinds of explanation might be suggested for these observations. First, the increase in poverty may be a result of ageing itself: for example, reaching the statutory retirement age causes a marked drop in most elderly people's incomes. However, it is harder to see why

---

[†] This chapter is a shortened version of a longer paper, the full version of which can be obtained from the authors on request.

age should be directly related to poverty in the years *after* retirement. Second, the relationship between age and poverty may be the consequence of other causal factors. In particular, as people move through their life course, they live in households of different composition, experience changing marital status, and have different sources of income. Since stage in life course is roughly correlated with age, the effect could be to generate an apparent relationship between age and poverty. If, for example, as one moves up the elderly age range, the proportion of married to non-married decreases, and if married couples are in general better off than the single or widowed elderly, one would expect to find that average income would decline with age.

A third kind of explanation for the relationship between income and age is that it is the result of a cohort effect: that is, older elderly people are poorer because they were born and spent their working lives during a different historical period from the 'young' elderly. Thus, for example, one of the major sources of income of elderly people is the occupational pension. The proportion of jobs with pension schemes has grown in the last twenty years, with the result that the 'young' elderly have a greater chance of benefiting from them than the older elderly. These three kinds of explanation, each of which will be explored in this chapter, are not mutually exclusive, but they do have different theoretical and policy implications.

For many elderly people, a statutory retirement pension is their major, if not their only resource. In addition, as they age, they are more likely to become disabled, and therefore to obtain more support from the state in the shape of free or subsidized health or social services. At the same time, some forms of state support are provided, not only on grounds of age or disability alone, but contingent on whether or not informal carers are seen as able to give assistance. The most likely potential informal carers are other members of the elderly person's household. Hence, the extent of provision of state support services may vary by household composition. The type of household in which the elderly person lives may, in its turn, be a function of the stage he or she has reached in the life course rather than of age *per se*. Thus, several factors may interact to affect in a complex way the distribution of income and the extent of service receipt by elderly people, and these too are explored below.

Data

The GHS is a nationally representative continuous survey of those living in private households. The data are drawn from the Surveys of 1979 and 1980 (OPCS 1981, 1982). In 1980 the GHS asked people aged 65 and over detailed questions on their level of disability, the nature and extent of help provided by informal carers, and their receipt of statutory services. The quality of the data, the high response rate, and the large size and representative nature of the sample make the GHS an invaluable source for examining a wide range of issues. However, because the sampling frame consists of private households only, the survey does not cover elderly people in institutional care — for example, those living in old people's homes and those who have been in hospital for more than six months. Because the proportion in such care rises with increasing age, the survey is more representative of those in the late 60s and early 70s than it is of the over-75s.

The 1980 Survey's section on the elderly was asked only of those aged 65 and over, and therefore tables in this chapter which are based on the 1980 data include only the subsample in this age band. Except where otherwise stated, the tables derived from the 1979 Survey include all those aged over the statutory retirement age at the time, 60 for women and 65 for men.

Resources and ageing

In 1979 (Figure 5.1), the median net income of households which included elderly people declined sharply with the age of the oldest member, from £43 per week for the 65–69 age-group to £32 for the 80-years-and-older group. 'Income' for the purpose of this figure was

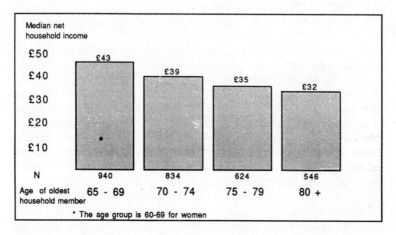

Figure 5.1 Net household income by age for all households containing at least one elderly member
Source: General Household Survey, 1979.

was calculated as the sum of the net (after tax) incomes from all sources for all the members of the household. However, single-person households with, for example, an income consisting only of a single person's state pension are much more likely to be found in the older age groups than in the younger ones. In other households there will be younger sons and daughters who are in paid work and this is more likely to be the case among those households in which the younger elderly live. In the younger age range, there may also be spouses who have not yet reached retirement age and are still in paid employment. It is possible that the steep age gradient observed in Figure 5.1 is mainly due to these factors.

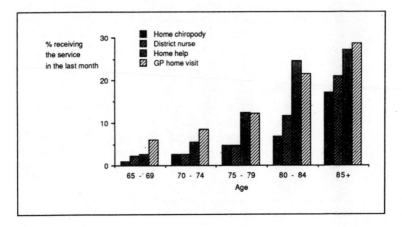

Figure 5.2 Service receipt in the last month, by age
Source: GHS, 1980.

The use of resources provided in kind by the state, such as health and welfare services, follows the reverse pattern, with usage increasing with age. As an example, Figure 5.2 shows that the likelihood of receiving home-help support in the last month rises from under 3 per cent in the 65–69 age-group to over a quarter for those aged over 80. A similar gradient is found for the receipt of district nurse visits, domiciliary chiropody, and general practitioner (GP) home visits. However, the simple interpretation that state service-provision varies proportionately with age may also be misleading. Factors such as degree of disability and whether the elderly person lives alone, with a spouse, or with younger household members may have a much stronger influence on service receipt than the age of the elderly person.

Table 5.1 shows that the kind of household in which elderly people live varies greatly by age. In the youngest age group, 65–69 years, most elderly people are living with their spouse, 37 per cent as one of a married couple whose partner is over 65, and 20 per cent with a partner under 65. In the next age range, 70–74, the most common arrangement is still living with an elderly spouse, but one in three elderly people are living by themselves, often because their spouse has died. The proportion of those living alone continues to climb until the 85-and-over age range, when the proportion living with others, either elderly people other than their spouse (11 per cent) or younger people, often their sons and daughters or other kin (29 per cent), becomes important.

Table 5.1 Type of household in which elderly people[a] live, by age (%)

Type of household	65–69	70–74	75–79	80–84	85+	All
Alone	23.7	31.8	41.8	51.3	48.2	33.6
Elderly married couple	37.0	44.1	36.7	23.8	12.5	36.2
Married couple, one spouse < 65	19.6	7.1	1.9	0.9	—	9.6
Two or more single elderly	2.7	4.4	4.6	6.0	10.5	4.3
Single elderly with single non-elderly(s)	5.0	4.7	6.1	8.0	14.7	6.0
Elderly couple with single non-elderly(s)	9.2	5.6	3.7	3.1	2.7	6.1
Elderly person or couple with non-elderly couple	2.8	2.5	5.2	6.9	11.3	4.1
All households	100.0 (1,656)	100.0 (1,258)	100.0 (887)	100.0 (450)	100.0 (257)	100.0 (4,508)
All	36.7	27.9	19.7	10.0	5.7	100.0

Source: GHS, 1980.
Note: a. Includes all those aged 65 and over and couples where one partner is aged over 65.
'Non-elderly' are those under 65 years old.
'Single' includes those never married, divorced and widowed.

The figures in Table 5.1 are from cross-sectional data, obtained in 1980, and could therefore be misleading as indicators of changes in households over time. However, Grundy (1986), using data from the OPCS Longitudinal Study which is based on a 1 per cent sample of the 1971 Census linked to records from the 1981 Census, reports a similar pattern. Her tables show that 16 per cent of the households containing a married couple with a partner aged 65–74 in 1971 and 23.5 per cent of married couple households with a partner aged 75 and over in 1971 had dissolved to a lone person household by 1981.

The fact that a relatively large number of elderly people, especially the 'old' elderly, live alone is a recent phenomenon (Table 5.2). The table documents a growth in the proportion of those living by themselves from around 10 per cent in 1945 to over one-third in 1980. The proportion living only with their spouse has also increased, from 30 per cent in 1945 to 44 per cent in 1980. These increases have been matched by a major decrease in the proportion living with others, from 60 per cent to 22 per cent. Similar changes are reported in the United States (Lee 1985). These changes in proportion are the more dramatic when considered alongside the growth in the absolute number of elderly people. In 1901 there were less than two million people over 65 in Britain, but by 1981 this had risen to about eight million (Henwood and Wicks 1985).

Table 5.2 Type of household of elderly people, 1945–80(%)

	1945[a]	1962	1976	1980
Living alone	10	22	30	34
Living with spouse	30	33	44	45
Living with others	60	44	27	22
	100	100	100	100

Source: from Dale *et al.* 1987
Note: a. These data are not nationally representative.

A variety of reasons have been put forward to explain these changes. There has been an increase in life expectancy, with the result that not only are there more elderly people, but there is also a greater likelihood that children will have left home long before the parents' death. In addition, children have tended to move out of the parental home at a younger age (Dale *et al.* 1987). Henwood and Wicks (1985) also cite the effects of the rising divorce rate. Lee (1985) argues from US data that many elderly people prefer independent living, but previously had to depend on the financial and other support of their children. With the advent of social security and pensions, elderly people are choosing to remain independent as long as they are able. Thompson and West (1984) also document the strong preference of many elderly to live alone compared with living with relatives or in an institution.

The great majority of the elderly living alone are women and this proportion increases with age from 79 per cent of those under 70 years of age to 86 per cent of those aged 80 or more (Table 5.3). This sex imbalance is primarily due to the shorter life-expectancy of men. In addition, however, women tend to marry men older than themselves. For both these reasons, there is a high likelihood that with advancing years wives will be widowed and will find themselves living alone.

Table 5.3 Percentage of women in 'elderly households'[a] by age and type of household

Type of household	65–69	70–74	75–79	80–84	85+	All
Alone	79	77	81	80	86	80
	(392)	(399)	(371)	(231)	(124)	(1,517)
Elderly married couple	59	49	43	28	41	50
	(613)	(555)	(325)	(107)	(32)	(1,632)
Married couple, one non-elderly spouse	20	15	6	25	–	19
	(324)	(89)	(17)	(4)	(0)	(434)
Two or more single elderly	77	64	78	70	85	74
	(44)	(55)	(41)	(27)	(27)	(194)
Single elderly with single non-elderly	69	75	80	78	92	77
	(87)	(61)	(55)	(37)	(38)	(278)
Elderly couple with single non-elderly	33	36	34	21	50	33
	(163)	(73)	(35)	(14)	(8)	(293)
Elderly person or couple with non-elderly couple	46	65	79	57	68	64
	(33)	(26)	(43)	(30)	(28)	(160)
All	54.5	56.9	63.6	62.7	78.5	59.1
	(1,656)	(1,258)	(887)	(453)	(257)	(4,508)

Source: GHS, 1980.
Note: a. Includes all those aged 65 and over and couples where one spouse is aged 65 and over. Age is that of the oldest member of the household.
'Non-elderly' are those aged under 65.
'Single' includes those never married, divorced, and widowed.
Base numbers in parentheses.

The income resources of the elderly

Comparisons between the incomes of age-groups, as in Figure 5.1, give only very rough indications of differences in disposable financial resources, for they do not fully take into account differences in household composition. A widely used measure which does to some extent standardize for the number of people in the household is 'Relative Net Resources' (RNR). RNR is the current weekly net household income in proportion to the DHSS supplementary-benefit level and takes the form of a percentage. This form of standardized income therefore controls for the size and composition of the household. Thus, for example, a household with an RNR value of 200 per cent has an income equal to twice the amount of benefit that it would be entitled to under the regulations of the time. Because households may include more than one of the 'assessment units' used by the DHSS to calculate rates of benefit, RNR is based on the sum of the entitlements of each assessment unit within the household.

It must be recognized, nevertheless, that RNR as a measure of relative resources has several defects. First, although interest on savings and investments is included, there is no available information on the value, for example, of shareholdings or investments such as paintings and jewellery. Second, it sets arbitrary amounts on the income needs of people of different ages and may underestimate the needs of children by comparison with adults (Berthoud 1985). It also fails to take into account regional differences in prices, and class-based spending customs (Kincaid 1979). Other general problems associated with using measures based on income include the difficulty of taking into account fringe benefits and payment-in-kind, gifts, and personal services (Townsend 1974). RNR indicates only the overall income resources of the whole household and does not assess their possibly unequal distribution within the household (Pahl 1983; Brannen and Wilson 1987). Of particular relevance is the fact that it may not allow sufficiently for the diseconomies of a single-person household.

As measured by RNR, the elderly are one of the poorest sub-groups. Figure 5.3 shows the level and distribution of RNR for a selection of household types which characterize stages of the life course (Dale 1987). It can be seen that the lone elderly had the lowest median income levels and also the most restricted range of income. This was because a substantial proportion were very heavily dependent upon the state for their income. Two-thirds of this group got over three-quarters of their income from state benefits and only 7 per cent had any earnings from employment. By contrast, median RNR levels were highest and the dispersion greatest where all adult members were of working age and there were no dependent children present.

The lone elderly group as a whole had a median RNR level of 110 per cent but as Table 5.4 shows, there were clear differences between men and women in every age-group. Men had a median value of 124 per cent, compared with 109 per cent for women. There was little variation in RNR with age for women living alone, but among men the youngest age-group, 65–69, had a considerably higher RNR level, 139 per cent, than the older groups (118 to 121 per cent). This was partly because a substantial proportion of these younger men (21 per cent) were still in paid work (Table 5.5). Although 15 per cent of the younger elderly women living alone were in paid work, this did not lift the income of the age-group to an appreciable extent, because of the poor wages they received. Younger elderly married couples were also better off than older couples, with income levels similar to those for the youngest age-group of lone elderly men, for the same reason. Among elderly couples where the oldest member was aged less than 70, as many as a third had at least one partner still doing some paid work.

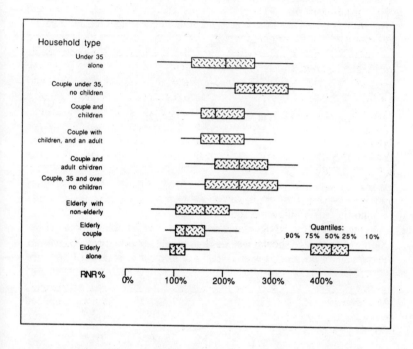

Figure 5.3 Relative Net Resources by household type, for household types characteristic of stages in the life course (from Dale, forthcoming)
Source: GHS 1979

A comparison of the characteristics of those in the highest and in the lowest income-quartile of each age category confirmed the central importance of the labour market in determining income in old age. Among the most well-off quartile of elderly people living alone (those with an RNR greater than 130 per cent), 19 per cent have some earned income, compared with 2 per cent in the lowest quartile (those with RNR less than 100 per cent). A similar pattern was found for elderly couples. Only 5 per cent of the lowest quartile had any income from paid employment compared with 45 per cent of the highest quartile.

In this connection, it should be noted that the proportion of elderly people in paid work has fallen very sharply since 1971. This has been the result of both the recession, which has promoted early retirement and redundancy, and the increasingly sharply drawn age of retirement.

Table 5.4 Median levels of RNR (relative net resources) by type of household and age of oldest member
Net income of household as a percentage of supplementary-benefit rate

Type of household	65–69[a]	70–74	75–79	80–84	All
Men alone	139	121	119	118	124
	(64)	(76)	(86)	(60)	(286)
Women alone	111	109	110	107	109
	(444)	(313)	(269)	(266)	(1,292)
Elderly married couples	130	132	125	120	129
	(278)	(315)	(150)	(92)	(835)
Two or more single elderly	124	108	103	124	110
	(12)	(27)	(32)	(34)	(105)

Source: GHS, 1979.
Note: a. Age range is 60–69 for women.
'Single' includes those never married, divorced, and widowed.
Base numbers in parentheses.

Table 5.5 Elderly households with someone in paid work by age of oldest member
Percentage of households with at least one member in paid work

Type of household	65–69[a]	70–74	75–79	80+	All
Men alone	21	9	5	3	9
	(67)	(80)	(93)	(67)	(307)
Women alone	15	4	3	0	7
	(467)	(330)	(283)	(283)	(1,363)
Elderly married couples	32	21	8	2	20
	(325)	(359)	(169)	(111)	(964)
Two or more single elderly	36	27	19	13	21
	(14)	(30)	(36)	(40)	(120)

Source: GHS, 1979.
Note: a. Age range is 60–69 for women.
'Single' includes those never married, divorced, and widowed.
Base numbers in parentheses.

As Townsend (1981) noted, retirement at pensionable age is now much more rigidly enforced, and 'old age pensioners' are assumed to have an economic-activity status very different from those of 'working age', irrespective of their state of health or capacity for work. The proportion of men aged 65–69 who are economically active has decreased particularly quickly, from 30 per cent in 1971 to only 11.4 per cent in 1986 (Table 5.6). The proportion of men aged 70 and over in the labour force has more than halved from 11 per cent to 5 per cent in the same time period. The shedding of older labour has also been a feature of the experience of the cohort just below the statutory retirement age, with male activity-rates in the 60–64 years age-group

Table 5.6 Percentage labour force activity rates, 1971–86

Men	1971	1976	1981	1986a
60–64	82.9	80.4	69.3	59.2
65–69	30.4	23.9	16.3	11.4
70+	10.9	8.0	6.5	4.7
Women				
55–59	50.9	54.3	53.4	51.9
60–64	28.8	26.9	23.3	21.2
65+	6.3	4.7	3.7	3.1

Source: Department of Employment (1985), Table 3, p. 259.
Note: a. Projection

falling from 83 per cent in 1971 to 60 per cent in 1986.

Amongst elderly women, there has also been a decrease in activity rates, but it is much less pronounced. The activity rate of women in the age-group just above the retirement age, 60–64, fell from 29 per cent in 1971 to 21 per cent in 1986. Moreover, the activity rate just before retirement, 55–59, has fractionally increased over this time period, so that nearly as many women as men are working as they approach the age of retirement. However, a much higher proportion of the women than the men are in part-time employment (Dale and Bamford 1987).

Current employment is one important factor affecting the disposable income of elderly people, but the influence of the labour market is still manifested, even in retirement, through the role of occupational pensions. As with employment, there are significant differences between men and women, and between household types, in the receipt of occupational pensions. In 1979 about 57 per cent of elderly married couples' incomes were supplemented by an occupational pension (usually arising from the husband's previous job) and the percentage for men living alone was much the same (Table 5.7). By contrast, only about 27 per cent of women living alone had an occupational pension. The difference is explained by the greater likelihood of men having held pensionable jobs, both because full-time jobs held by men were more likely to have pension rights than women's, and because, before the age of retirement, a majority of older women had either no paid job or a part-time job with no pension provision.

Overlaying these gender differences, there is a cohort effect. The older age-groups were somewhat less likely than the younger ones to have an occupational pension. Thus, for example, the proportion of men living alone who received a pension rose from 52 per cent at 80 years and over, to 61 per cent for those aged 65–69, reflecting the growth in provision of occupational pensions between the early sixties when the oldest age-group

Table 5.7 Percentage of elderly households with at least one member receiving an occupational pension, by age of oldest person

Type of household	65–69[a]	70–74	75–79	80+	All
Men alone	61	59	57	52	65
	(64)	(76)	(86)	(60)	(286)
Women alone	32	28	27	15	27
	(444)	(313)	(269)	(266)	(1,292)
Elderly married	57	61	56	50	57
couples	(278)	(315)	(150)	(92)	(835)
Two or more	58	48	50	59	53
single elderly	(12)	(27)	(32)	(34)	(105)

Source: GHS, 1979.
Note: a. Age range is 60–69 for women.
'Single' includes those never married, divorced, and widowed.
Base numbers in parentheses.

left the labour force and the late seventies when the most recently retired left. The growth in occupational pension provision for women was even more marked with more than double the proportion of 60–69 year olds having them (32 per cent) compared with the over-80s (15 per cent). Re-entry into the labour force after child-rearing was less usual for the older group than for the younger (Martin and Roberts 1984) and therefore fewer would have had pensionable paid employment in the years before retirement.

Among elderly people living alone, 63 per cent of the highest quartile of RNR had occupational pensions, compared with 10 per cent of those in the lowest quartile, underlining the importance of such pensions in determining income at this age. In the highest quartile, the mean age was 72 and 30 per cent were men. In the lowest quartile, the mean age was only slightly older, 74, and 16 per cent were men. There was a similar lack of relationship between age and receipt of an occupational pension in the elderly married couple household group, where 74 per cent of those in the highest quartile had occupational pensions and the mean age of the older partner was 72, while only 27 per cent of those in the lowest quartile had occupational pensions and the mean age of the oldest partner was 73.

Although at first sight, therefore, it seems that there was a strong age-related gradient in the overall net income of elderly people, the effect was largely accounted for by the dissolution of married-couple households when husbands died, leaving widows significantly worse off not only than married couples, but also than men living on their own. The higher income of married couples and men living alone was the combined result of the continued involvement of men in the labour market after the statutory retirement age, although this had decreased sharply over the previous few years, and of the receipt of occupational pensions. Despite the fact that the incomes of elderly married couples and of men living alone were considerably higher than that of elderly women living alone, both groups were near to the bottom of the distribution of income when compared with households not including elderly people.

The receipt of statutory services

State provision is important for many elderly people, not only because they have to rely on a retirement or supplementary pension in the absence of income from employment or from an occupational pension, but also because they need the health and social services provided by the welfare state. However, state support varies in a complex way according to the age of the elderly person, the extent of his or her disability, the type of household lived in, and the informal support available. As we shall demonstrate, the effect of the interaction of these various factors is that for some kinds of service, the elderly living alone obtain more support from the state than those living in other types of household. At the same time, in all households, the state provides little support compared with that forthcoming from other carers, particularly from other members of the elderly person's household.

Not unnaturally, the amount of statutory health and social services which individuals receive depends in part on the level of their need. Elderly people's 'need' for support is difficult to measure directly, but a reasonable indicator can be obtained by asking them about their capacity to perform a range of daily living activities and self-care tasks, and about their mobility. Their answers can be used to construct an index of functional disability (Townsend and Wedderburn 1965; Bebbington and Davies 1983; Arber *et al.* 1988). When this was done with the GHS 1980 data, half the elderly people (49 per cent) had no disability and a quarter some slight disability (26 per cent). About 11 per cent were 'severely disabled', most of them having difficulty or requiring help in getting up stairs and around the house and in having a bath.

As might be expected, the prevalence of disability varied greatly with age. Only 5 per cent of people under 70, but more than 40 per cent of those over 85, were classified as severely disabled (Table 5.8). The proportion severely disabled also differed with gender, women living alone being considerably more likely to be disabled than men living alone, at all ages. It also differed with the type of household in which elderly people lived, particularly among those aged 85 and over. Within this oldest group, those living alone or with a spouse alone were considerably less likely to be severely disabled than those living with younger kin or with other elderly people. These findings suggest that disability levels help to determine the type of household in which elderly people live.

If statutory support-services were channelled to those who were the

Table 5.8 Percentage of 'severely disabled' elderly people (a score of 6 and above on an index of functional disability)[a] by age and type of household

Type of household	65–69	70–74	75–79	80–84	85+	All
Man alone	2	2	6	13	29	6
	(81)	(89)	(68)	(45)	(17)	(300)
Woman alone	5	9	14	24	33	14
	(310)	(300)	(293)	(181)	(99)	(1,183)
Elderly[b] married	4)	7	10	22	35	7
couple	(906)	(615)	(330)	(107)	(29)	(1,987)
Two or more	10	12	20	22	48	19
single elderly	(41)	(52)	(37)	(23)	(25)	(178)
Elderly with single	7	9	9	21	56	13
non-elderly(s)	(239)	(123)	(89)	(47)	(41)	(539)
Elderly with	10	20	8	32	46	22
non-elderly couple	(29)	(25)	(39)	(28)	(26)	(147)
All	4.7	8.0	11.2	22.7	41.0	10.7
	(1,606)	(1,204)	(856)	(431)	(237)	(4,334)

Source: GHS, 1980.
Note: a. Defined in Evandrou *et al*. 1986.
     b. Includes those married to a spouse aged less than 65 years.
'Non-elderly' are those under 65 years old.
'Single' includes those never married, divorced, and widowed.
Base numbers in parentheses.

most disabled, one would expect from these results to find that the elderly living with others would obtain more of them than elderly married couples or the elderly living alone. In fact, as Table 5.9 indicates, the situation in 1980 was very different in regard to two tasks for which older people often need assistance — shopping and cutting toe-nails. The pattern of sources of help with shopping shown in the table was also typical of that for a range of other domestic and personal house-care tasks, including cooking, washing, and bathing (Evandrou *et al.* 1986).

Some 14 per cent of the 1980 GHS sample aged over 65 could not do their shopping themselves and 28 per cent could not cut their own toe-nails (OPCS 1982). Table 5.9 demonstrates that the state provided minimal help with shopping except to those living alone. Most of them (76 per cent) received help from relatives, friends, and neighbours. The state services did, however, make a greater contribution than did informal carers to chiropody when that was needed, in all types of household.

These data suggest that the state's contribution of resources to elderly households through the provision of support services is, for most services, not substantial and that it varies with the type of household. However, since the proportion who are disabled in different types of household also varies, it is necessary to see whether the differences in state provision remain after the level of disability has been controlled. This is done

Table 5.9 Usual source of help by those requiring some help with (a) shopping and (b) cutting toe-nails by type of household (percentage receiving help)
(a) Shopping

Source of help			Type of household		
				Elderly with younger household members	
	Alone	Married couple	Two or more elderly	Alone	Married
In household					
Spouse	—	80	—	—	53
Other	—	—	78	90	39
Outside household					
Child	38	7	3	4	6
Other	18	5	16	1	1
Friend or neighbour	20	6	3	4	1
Social or medical service	21	2	0	1	0
Paid help	3	0	0	0	0
	100	100	100	100	100
	(298)	(37)	(253)	(163)	(70)

(b) Cutting toe-nails

	Alone	Married couple	Two or more elderly	Alone	Married
In household					
Spouse	—	34	—	—	28
Other	—	—	22	34	20
Outside household					
Child	8	4	2	4	2
Other relative	3	1	0	1	2
Friend or neighbour	3	1	0	1	0
Social or medical service	86	60	76	60	48
Paid help	0	0	0	0	0
	100	100	100	100	100
	(486)	(439)	(63)	(156)	(80)

Source: GHS, 1980.

by using a logit analysis (Arber *et al.* (forthcoming) discuss the analysis in more detail). Table 5.10 shows odds ratios for the receipt of three statutory services, for different types of household, after controlling for disability, in each case comparing the level of service received with that for elderly married people. An elderly man living alone, for example, was 5.74 times more likely to have had a home-help visit during the previous month than an elderly couple, after allowing for the different average disability levels of the two types of household.

Elderly people living alone received very much more assistance from home helps than any other type of household. The odds ratio shows that

Table 5.10 Receipt of statutory services at home in the last month
Odds ratios, compared with the level of receipt by the husband of elderly married couples, controlling for disability

Type of household	Home help	Chiropodist's home visit	GP home visit	N
Man alone	5.74	2.71	1.34	(300)
Woman alone	5.28	2.23	1.35	(1,172)
Elderly married couple				
husband ⎤		1.00	1.00	(777)
wife ⎦	1.00	1.30	0.90	(776)
Two or more				
single elderly	1.31	2.21	0.94	(178)
Elderly with				
non-elderly				
male(s)	0.75	1.80	1.36	(151)
female(s)	0.81	1.67	0.84	(102)
Married elderly[a] with				
single non-elderly	—	1.52	1.11	(260)
Elderly with non-				
elderly spouse	0.24	0.19	0.90	(419)
Elderly with non-				
elderly married couple				
or lone parent	0.22	1.57	1.07	(147)

Source: GHS, 1980.

Note: a. Includes couples where one partner is under 65.
'Non-elderly' are those under 65 years old.
'Single' includes those never married, divorced, and widowed.

this was the case even after taking into account the fact that those living alone tended to be more disabled than elderly married couples, and therefore in greater need of such help. Elderly people living with other, younger people were much less likely to have had a home-help visit in the last month than households containing only elderly people. Those who lived with a younger married couple were about five times less likely to receive a home-help visit than an elderly married couple. It is fair to conclude, therefore, that statutory services were provided to a much greater extent to those who have no one else to call upon within the household than to those who live with others.

The picture for home visits from a GP was very different, with a much smaller range of variation between types of household. The situation for chiropody at home was mid-way between that for the receipt of home help and GP visits, with the ratio for elderly men living alone being 2.7 times higher than for elderly married men. The three services differ in their 'substitutability' — that is, the degree to which informal carers (other household members, relatives, and friends) are expected to be able to substitute for the services which might be provided by formal carers (paid professionals) (Arber *et al.* 1988). Of the three, home helps are the most and GP visits the least substitutable, and the pattern of receipt of statutory services varies accordingly. In each case it is elderly people living alone who obtain the most support from the state, and among them men receive slightly more than women.

The conclusions which can be drawn from this examination of the use of state-funded welfare services by elderly people are that the 'older' among them obtain much more help than the 'younger', primarily because, on average, they are much more disabled. However, there is also a strong, independent effect of the type of household in which the elderly person lives. Hence, the overall use of state-support services depends on the combination of the effects of disability, the type of household, and the substitutability of the service. Elderly people living alone are more likely to receive substitutable state-funded services than those living in other types of household with comparable levels of disability. The latter — that is, those living with spouses and with younger people — are most likely to obtain support from those living with them and little from the state.

Resources and the life course

This analysis has shown that the relationship between resources and age is more complex than is immediately apparent. After distinguishing different types of household in terms of their composition and structure, variation in income with age *within* each household type is not great. On the other hand, different types of household have very different incomes, even after standardizing for the number of people in the household and including all sources of income: households of elderly women living alone are poorer than other types of household. In short, the overall apparent relationship between income and age is accounted for primarily by the changing proportions of types of household with age. While married couples are the most common type amongst the under 75s, women alone are the most common type of household among the over-75 age-group.

Those differences in income with age which remain after considering each type of household separately can mainly be explained in terms of two factors. First, in households consisting of elderly married couples, one of the spouses may still be working and contributing to the household income. Second, the recent increase in occupational pension schemes causes a 'cohort' effect. The older groups are less likely to have contributed to such a scheme while they were in the labour force, and are therefore less likely to have an occupational pension.

In addition to income from benefits and pensions, elderly households also receive a considerable amount of services in kind, largely at no cost to themselves, mainly from relatives but also from the statutory health and social services. The amount of support obtained from statutory services depends on the elderly person's degree of disability but also on the type of household in which he or she lives. Disability increases with age, and also varies between those living in different types of household: women living alone and those living with younger married couples are particularly likely to be severely disabled. There are great differences in the contribution which statutory services make to supporting households which include elderly people: those living alone receive the most, and those in households with younger people the least.

While it is true, as Table 5.1 showed, that the distribution of elderly people between different types of household is strongly correlated to their age, the link between household type and age is not a simple causal one. The type of household lived in is better considered a consequence of the stage they have reached in their life course than of their age *per se* (Dale 1987). Similarly, the resources of elderly people are more clearly explained in terms of their stage of life than of their age. Figure 5.4 summarizes some of the data presented in this chapter in these terms. It represents all households which contain an elderly person.

One can distinguish a typical trajectory — shown moving down from the upper left of the figure — as married couples reach the statutory retirement-age. Following the cessation of earnings, their income drops sharply, from a median value of 240 per cent RNR to about 130 per cent. Some 31 per cent of elderly households consist of such married couples.

The trajectory continues in a downward direction with the death of a spouse, most likely the husband, and the formation of a single-person household. Some 42 per cent of households containing an elderly person consist of a lone woman. Income for this group is very low, but receipt of statutory support-services is relatively great; for example, those living alone receive five times more services than married couples. A few elderly people, as they get older and more disabled, join the households of younger kin. They are shown moving up the figure and their RNR increases. Although his or her *personal* income will not increase, the elderly person's situation appears to be considerably improved because the standardized income of the household will be greater and the younger household members will provide much of the substitutable care which would otherwise have been obtained from the health and social services. Whether this is truly an improvement will depend on factors such as the value the elderly person places on independence (Thompson and West 1984) and the distribution of resources within the household.

The slightly higher RNR levels for elderly married couples and for men living alone than for women living alone are because the women have less income from paid employment and from occupational pensions. The importance of these sources of income has implications for the

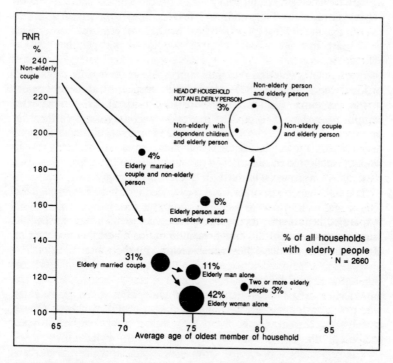

Figure 5.4 Life course trajectory: type of household on axes of the age of the oldest member of the household and the median household RNR
Source:GHS 1980.

income in old age of men and women who are now in their fifties and who are faced with long-term unemployment or early retirement. The groups at the higher points on the diagram — that is, those with higher median levels of RNR — consist of households in which the elderly live with younger people and it is one or more of the younger members who own or rent the home. These households have higher median levels of RNR mainly as a result of the income from paid employment of one or more of these younger household members.

The decline in labour market participation of men in particular from 55 years onwards (Laczko and Walker, 1985;. Laczko *et al.*, forthcoming) seems to imply that it will become increasingly difficult for those over retirement age to obtain any paid work with which to supplement their pension. Unemployment levels amongst school-leavers are such that many of the casual and part-time jobs once filled by those of retirement age are now being taken by young people. Although occupational pension schemes are increasingly common, levels of payment are often linked to earnings in the most recent years of work. Furthermore, women who work part-time are often ineligible to join an occupational-pension scheme.

For women, who make up the majority of the increasing proportion of lone elderly people, there seems little prospect of an improvement in their economic position unless there is a considerable rise in the basic statutory pension. The current moves to encourage still further the provision of private occupational-pensions in preference to state schemes may serve only to emphasize the inequalities between some elderly people who are supported by one or even two occupational pensions, and those, particularly widows, who have only their state pension.

The 'U'-shaped resources trajectory traced in Figure 5.4 through the later stages of life, first as a couple, then as a widow living alone, and then with other younger people is only one hypothetical trajectory. During this trajectory, some move into institutional care and therefore out of the population we have been considering. Furthermore, the detailed picture is much more complicated than the trajectory might suggest. As Figure 5.4 shows, for example, 6 per cent of elderly households include an elderly married couple with another adult, often a son or daughter who has never left the parental home, and 3 per cent contain two or more elderly, non-married people. Neither these, nor a variety of other types of household fit into the stereotypical trajectory through the life course.

Figure 5.4 does, however, show clearly the particular income disadvantage of elderly people living alone. They receive relatively more health and social services but, under the current funding arrangements and level of provision, these services have great difficulty in meeting existing demands upon them. If the number of elderly people living alone increases, as projections suggest (Henwood and Wicks 1985), and if the value of occupational pensions is reduced and jobs to supplement state benefits become rarer, the prospect for the standard of living of elderly people as a whole is not encouraging.

Acknowledgements

We thank the Office of Population Censuses and Surveys (OPCS) for their support and for permission to use the General Household Survey, and the ESRC Data Archive for their continuing help. The research was funded by the Economic and Social Research Council, Grant G0125003, as part of the Ageing Initiative. The ESRC also provided support for the preparation of the GHS into SPSS and SIR files (Grant HR8360).

This chapter is the combined effort of all those involved in the Ageing Initiative project, 'Employment and Ageing: the older worker, and the impact of elderly relatives in the household' at the University of Surrey. Much of the background to the paper draws upon work by Maria Evandrou and Frank Laczko, research officers on the project. The work on income and old age is by Angela Dale, while that on service provision has mainly been carried out by Sara Arber. The paper was written by Nigel Gilbert in collaboration with the other main authors. It was first presented at the ESRC Workshop on Ageing at the University of Surrey, September 1986. This version has benefited greatly from the comments of Margot Jefferys.

References

Arber, S. Gilbert, G.N. and Evandrou, M. (1988) 'Gender, household composition and receipt of domiciliary services by elderly disabled people', *Journal of Social Policy* 17 (2): 153–75.

Bebbington, A. and Davies, B. (1983) 'Equity and efficiency in the allocation of personal social services', *Journal of Social Policy* 12:309–30.

Berthoud, R. (1985) *The Examination of Social Security*, London: Policy Studies Institute.

Brannen,J. and Wilson, G. (eds) (1987) *Give and Take in Families. Studies in Resource Distribution*, London: George Allen & Unwin.

Cantor, M. (1979) 'Neighbours and friends: an overlooked resource in the informal support system', *Research on Ageing* 1: 434–63.

Dale, A. (1987) 'The effects of life-cycle on three dimensions of stratification', in A. Bryman *et al.* (eds) *Life Cycle Perspectives*, London: Macmillan.

Dale, A. and Bamford, C. (1987) 'Older workers and the peripheralisation of the workforce — the erosion of gender differences', University of Surrey, mimeo.

Dale, A. Evandrou, M., and Arber, S. (1987) 'The household structure of the elderly in Britain', *Journal of Social Policy* 7 (1).

Department of Employment (1985) 'Labour force outlook for Great Britain', *Employment Gazette* July: 255–60.

Evandrou, M., Arber, S. Dale, A., and Gilbert, G.N. (1986) 'Who cares for the elderly? Family care provision and receipt of statutory services', in C. Phillipson, M. Bernard, and P. Strang (eds) *Dependency and Interdependency in Old Age: Theoretical Perspectives and Policy Alternatives*, London: Croom Helm.

Grundy, E. (1986) 'Age related changes in later life', Conference on Population Research in Britain, University of East Anglia, September.

Henwood, M., and Wicks, M. (1985) 'Community care, family trends and social change', *Quarterly Journal of Social Affairs* 1: 357–71.

Kincaid, J. (1979) 'Poverty in the welfare state', in J. Irvine, I. Miles and J. Evans (eds) *Demystifying Social Statistics*, London: Pluto Press, pp. 212–21

Laczko, F. and Walker, A. (1985) 'Excluding older workers from the labour force: early retirement policies in Britain, France and Sweden', in *The Yearbook of Social Policy 1984-5*, London: Routledge.

Laczko, F., Dale, A., Arber, S., and Gilbert, G.N. (forthcoming) 'Early retirement in a period of high unemployment', *Journal of Social Policy*.

Layard, R., Piachaud, D., and Stewart, M. (1978) *The Causes of Poverty*, Royal Commission on the Distribution of Income and Wealth, London: HMSO.

Lee, G.R. (1985) 'Kinship and social support of the elderly: the case of the United States', *Ageing and Society* 5: 19–38.

Martin, J. and Roberts, C. (1984) *Women and Employment: A Lifetime Perspective*, London: HMSO.

Office of Population Censuses and Surveys (OPCS) (1981) *General Household Survey*, 1979, London: HMSO.

Office of Population Censuses and Surveys (1982) *General Household Survey*, 1980, London: HMSO.

Pahl, J. (1983) 'The allocation of money and the structuring of inequality within marriage', *Sociological Review* 31: 237–62.

Shanas, E., Townsend, P., Wedderburn, D., Friis, H., Milhof, P., and Stenhouwer, J. (1968) *Old People in three industrial societies*, London: Routledge & Kegan Paul.

Taylor, R., and Ford, G. (1983) 'Inequalities in old age: an examination of age, sex and class differences in a sample of community elderly', *Ageing and Society* 4: 183–208.

Thompson, C. and West, P. (1984) 'The public appeal of sheltered housing', *Ageing and Society* 4: 305–26.

Townsend, P. (1974) 'Poverty as relative deprivation: resources and style of living', in D. Wedderburn (ed.) *Poverty, Inequality and Class Structure*, Cambridge: Cambridge University Press, pp. 15–42.

Townsend, P. (1979) *Poverty in the United Kingdom*, Harmondsworth: Penguin.

Townsend, P. (1981) 'The structured dependency of the elderly: a creation of social policy in the twentieth century', *Ageing and society* 1: 5–28.

Townsend P. and Wedderburn, D. (1965) *The Aged in the Welfare State*, G. Bell and Sons.

Walker, A. (1980) 'The social creation of poverty and dependency in old age' *Journal of Social Policy* 9; 49–75.

Victor, C. and Evandrou, M. (1986) 'Social class and the elderly', Annual Conference of the British Sociological Association, Loughborough, March.

Chapter six

Income Inequality in Later Life

Christina R. Victor

Introduction

Old age is a stage in the life cycle about which there are numerous stereotypes. It is commonly believed that the elderly live socially isolated existences, beset with health problems and experiencing considerable emotional stress. Another popular stereotype is that the elderly population constitutes a homogeneous social group. This reflects the commonly held view of old age as a great leveller. Consequently, older people are perceived, by both the general public and many social researchers, as all being alike.

By convention the elderly population in Britain is usually defined as that fraction of the total population entitled to the state retirement-pension — 60 years for women and 65 years for men. This broad phase of the life cycle covers an age range of thirty years and more. Few social researchers would combine the 20–49 year olds in a single social category. Yet this is what many do unthinkingly when they use the term 'the elderly'. Recently social gerontologists have begun to deconstruct the single social category 'the old' into groups defined in terms of age, household composition, ethnic origin, and gender.

One of the most enduring stereotypes of old age is its characterization as a time of poverty and great deprivation. The association of old age with poverty is not a recent phenomenon. Many of the Victorian social researchers and reformers commented on the extreme poverty and privation which the elderly population endured. Indeed, such is the strength and durability of the assumed relationship between old age and poverty that the latter is now perceived as a 'natural' part of ageing. Recent debates about the income of older people, however, have concentrated upon examining their position relative to other members of society (Fiegehen 1986). This threatens to lead to the development of a new stereotype representing later life as a time of affluence.

In this chapter I examine the distribution of incomes within the elderly

115

population in 1980, and in particular the sources from which they were derived.

Sources of income in later life

Older people drew their income from four major sources: pensions, savings, earnings from employment, and gifts from relatives and friends. Pensions were derived from two major sources: previous employers, when they were known as occupational pensions, and the state.

Occupational pensions

Occupational pensions were arranged by either individual employers, or groups of employers. The pension level was usually based upon the length of time the individual had worked for the employer and the amount of final earnings. Under most arrangements the individual received a fraction of the salary received at the time of retirement. Occupational pensions have a long tradition in Britain where the very first pensions were occupationally based rather than state-provided. Initially they were used as a method of attracting and retaining staff in occupations for which a lengthy training was required. However, it has been alleged that they have also been used as a means of ridding the work-force of older workers (Phillipson 1982).

In 1980, many occupational pension schemes did not cover part-time workers, most of whom were women, and were most generous to those in the highest-paid occupations. They did not cover all the working population. In public-sector employment most full-time employees were included in a scheme; but, in the private sector, only about 50 per cent of males and 30 per cent of females were covered (Groves 1986). In all, 63 per cent of full-time male employees and 56 per cent of women were members of an occupational pension scheme in 1985 (OPCS 1986). The coverage of part-time workers was considerably lower.

Perhaps the most significant criticism of current British occupational pension schemes is that they are not 'occupational' in the true sense of the term; rather, they are employer-, not occupationally based. A shop assistant who changed her job in 1980 from Woolworths to Marks and Spencer, for example, had not changed her occupation but had changed her employer. As a result she would have changed her pension scheme membership because there was no single scheme for shop assistants. Consequently, she would have become an early leaver from one pension scheme and a new entrant to another. Occupational pensions, other than those operating in the public sector, tended then to penalize those who frequently changed jobs.

State income-support in later life

The current pattern of state income-support for later life is a two-tier system whose origins lie in the state social security scheme proposed by Beveridge in the 1940s. The main component of the state system is a compulsory system of national insurance to provide protection against what Beveridge saw as the major causes of poverty; old age, unemployment, widowhood, and sickness. Supplementing this is a 'safety net' of means-tested assistance called, successively, National Assistance, Supplementary Benefit, and Income Support, which provides for those inadequately covered by the insurance scheme.

The underlying premiss of the Beveridge plan was that of universality of coverage. All adults should be afforded protection against the major causes of poverty and income interruption via a system of compulsory national insurance. The only criterion for eligibility for benefits was to be contributions to the insurance fund. The retirement-pension under the scheme is payable to women at age 60 and men at age 65 provided that they have retired from employment. It is a flat-rate benefit paid automatically to those with the appropriate contributions record who have retired from work. In 1984–5, 9.3 million elderly people received this pension at a cost of £15.3 billion (DHSS 1984). The level at which the retirement pension is paid is set annually by Parliament. Since 1980, increases in the pension have been linked to increases in wages. Previously the pension level had been linked to increases in wages or prices, whichever was the larger. According to Walker (1986), the result of this change in the method of setting the pension level was to decrease the real income of pensioners by 12 per cent between 1980 and 1985. Although the absolute value of the pension in real terms has increased since 1948, its value as a fraction of the average earnings of a male manual worker rose only slightly from 19.1 per cent in 1948 to 22.9 per cent in 1983 (DHSS 1984).

Beveridge assumed that as the coverage of the insurance scheme increased, the need for means-tested income support for older people would gradually diminish. He foresaw a situation in which National Assistance, as these latter types of benefits were then called, would be phased out. In the event, however, there has been an increase in the kinds of means-tested benefits available and in the number and proportion of older people dependent on them. In 1948 one million claims for National Assistance were made by pensioners compared with 5,482,137 in 1984. During the same period the number of pensioners increased from 6.7 million to 9.7 million. Means-tested benefits provided 11 per cent of pensioners' incomes in 1984–5, an increase of 3 per cent over the situation in 1951 (ibid.).

There were over forty such benefits available in 1980 and responsibility for their administration was divided between national and local government. The most important of these benefits was Supplementary Benefit. Supplementary Pension (SP) was the component of the system relevant to older people. It was paid to pensioners who, after undergoing a means test, could demonstrate that their income was below a specified level and any capital assets they possessed below a prescribed amount.

The effectiveness of means testing as a way of targeting money to those most in need is limited because of the persistent and deep-rooted problem of low take-up. Means-tested benefits, with the exception of student grants, consistently fail to be claimed by all those entitled to the benefit. In 1983, 67 per cent of eligible pensioners were in receipt of supplementary pension. Some 790,000 elderly were not receiving the benefit, leaving £233 million allocated for the year unclaimed: an average payment of £5.60 a week (Bradshaw 1985). It seems likely that, at that time too, more than 20 per cent of older people entitled to housing benefit were not receiving it.

Take-up encompasses two specific dimensions (Beltram 1984). First, there is the non-claiming of benefits by those eligible for them. An example of this would be a pensioner with low income failing to claim entitlement to supplementary pension. The second involves under-claiming and includes those who, although receiving a particular benefit, might not be getting their complete entitlement. Thus, for example, a pensioner might be receiving a flat-rate supplementary pension but not the heating addition to which she was entitled. There are no data available about the extent of the under-claiming of benefits by older people (or any other claimant group), but in 1980 it was likely to be significant.

Method

In order to investigate the distribution of income within the elderly population, a secondary analysis of the 1980 General Household Survey (GHS) was undertaken. Information on 4,553 people aged 65 years and over was included in the data-set for that year. It also included a series of supplementary questions concerning disability, the provision of informal care, and use of community services which were asked only of those aged 65 years and over. Standard information on social class, tenure, life-style, and income was also collected.

The GHS regularly collects information upon income and is a well validated and reliable source of such data. Complete information on income was obtained from 4,038 of the 4,553 elderly people who participated in the survey, partial income data were obtained from the remainder. Subjects for whom only partial income data were available were included in some parts of the analysis. The result was that the range between minimum and maximum incomes is probably exaggerated since some very low total incomes were included in the analysis.

A variety of income indices may be calculated from the GHS: for example, information was available about the total income of the individual, of the family unit, and of the household. In each case the totals are calculated by summing the income from four major sources; state pensions/benefits, earnings from employment, occupational pensions, and unearned income. This last source includes rent from property, and interest from investments in banks, building societies, and other similar sources. The GHS does not record transfers of income between family members nor, not surprisingly, transactions in the 'black economy'. Consequently GHS data probably underestimate total incomes. This chapter considers the incomes of individuals and of households, on the assumption that there were no substantial differences between household and family-unit income.

Total income

Table 6.1 shows the total weekly household and individual income of older people in Britain in 1980. To put these and subsequent data into context, the average male manual worker's wage in 1980 was approximately £100 a week. The table illustrates the wide range of incomes recorded for older people included in the GHS: individual incomes varied from a few pence a week, reflecting the influence of incomplete data obtained for some individuals, to £770, or £40,000 per annum. Similar variations characterized total household income.

Table 6.1 Income measures for elderly people — weekly income

	Total individual income	*Total household income*
Mean	£34.84	£65.21
Median	£29.78	£47.15
Maximum	£717.30	£717.30
N	4,138	4,368

Source: GHS, 1980

The table also serves to highlight one of the major problems in presenting data on income distribution for older age-groups: the selection of the appropriate summary statistic. Two measures of central tendency are given in Table 6.1: the arithmetic mean and the median. The arithmetic mean gives a higher figure than the median; the mean weekly household income was £53.16p compared with the median figure of £42.25p. In subsequent analysis the median income is used, as this statistic takes into account the range of income distributions and is not artificially inflated or deflated by the presence of extreme income levels.

Median total household income, classified by the age and sex of the head of the household, shows substantial age-based inequalities (Table 6.2). As the age of the head of the household increased, income levels declined. The median income for households headed by men aged 80 and over was £13 a week less than that for households headed by men aged 65–69. Similarly, households headed by women aged 80 and over had a median weekly income which was £9 a week less than that of households headed by women aged 65–69. The general age-related pattern was further overlaid by a marked gender difference. At all ages, households headed by women had a lower median income than those headed by men. The difference was largest for the 65–69 age-group. Households headed by men of this age had a weekly income which was £13 larger than that of households headed by women. The difference decreased as the age of the household head increased independent of changes in the size of households. However, even in the oldest age-group, the weekly income of households headed by women was £7 a week less than households headed by men of the same age.

Table 6.2 Median weekly household income by age and sex of head of household (to nearest £)

Age-group	Male	Female
65–69	£63	£49
70–74	£52	43
75–79	£48	£38
80+	£47	£36

Source: GHS, 1980.

Using the main life-time occupation of the head or her spouse, households were classified into the traditional five-fold social-class typology. There are problems in applying this classification to older people (Victor and Evandrou 1987), and especially to households headed by widowed women who are classified according to the job held by their spouse. Leaving aside these conceptual and practical difficulties, it is clear that social class was an important source of income differentiation (Table 6.3). For households headed by men there was a clear tendency for weekly income to diminish from Social Classes 1 or 2 to Social Classes 4 or 5. In such households those categorized by the head as belonging to professional and managerial occupation groups had a median income 60 per cent higher than their counterparts from the unskilled and semi-skilled groups. The differential between manual and non-manual workers was independent of age.

Table 6.3 Median individual weekly income by age, sex, and social class of head (to nearest £)

		1 & 2 £ N	3n £ N	3m £ N	4 & 5 £ N
		Social class			
65-69	M	57 (121)	47 (134)	35 (262)	35 (171)
	F	30 (51)	24 (247)	23 (78)	23 (396)
70-74	M	43 (92)	36 (86)	32 (185)	33 (136)
	F	27 (41)	24 (185)	25 (71)	26 (305)
75-79	M	40 (68)	34 (45)	30 (113)	31 (69)
	F	29 (34)	27 (142)	26 (53)	28 (243)
80+	M	36 (30)	35 (33)	30 (71)	28 (58)
	F	31 (20)	28 (106)	29 (55)	29 (181)

Source: GHS, 1980.

The position is rather more complex for households headed by women. With the exception of the youngest age-group, there was no clear trend for their income to vary substantially with social class. Presumably this reflects the problem of classifying widows on the basis of their husband's occupation, a classification which is both indirect and retrospective. It cannot be taken to imply that social class was not a factor of importance in the lives of older women.

I now examine the distribution of income from different sources in the GHS sample.

National Insurance Retirement Pension

The National Insurance Retirement Pension, known colloquially as the 'old age pension', was received by the majority, 95 per cent, of the sample. Simple receipt did not vary significantly with either age, social class, or gender. The essentially flat-rate nature of this benefit was reflected in the similarity of the mean (£22.74) and median (£23.54) weekly payments and the lack of variation with age, sex, or social class in the median weekly payment received. An earnings-related supplement payable on this pension was introduced in 1961, but as it was not inflation proofed it did not make any significant impact on the national insurance pension level for the majority of recipients.

Occupational pensions

Occupational pensions were received by 31 per cent of the GHS sample. The receipt varied markedly by sex and age: men were more likely to receive it than women and the younger than the older (Table 6.4). The cohort effect reflected a substantial recent increase in the number of people entitled to such a pension. The lower prevalence amongst women reflected both their lower overall labour market participation rate compared with men, and its concentration in jobs which did not have occupational pension schemes. In addition to the age and gender effects, social class also exerted an influence on the receipt of this pension. For each age-group those from non-manual occupations were more likely to receive this type of pension than manual workers.

Table 6.4 Percentages of elderly persons receiving occupational pensions by social class, age, and gender

Social Class	Age									
	65–69		70–74		75–79		80+		All ages	
	M	F	M	F	M	F	M	F	M	F
I & II	76	28	68	17	53	41	68	36	64	24
IIIn	64	23	60	25	53	33	40	25	52	25
IIIm	55	17	44	17	47	11	56	25	48	17
IV & V	55	11	46	16	39	16	34	15	46	14
All Classes	57	16	48	17	44	21	43	18	51	18
N	(698)	(809)	(507)	(611)	(298)	(476)	(195)	(367)	(1,698)	(2,263)

Source: GHS, 1980.

There was a great range in the amount of occupational pension received (Table 6.5). The mean weekly pension payment was £107.56 a week compared with the median value of £15 a week. The maximum pension received was £750 a week (or an annual income of £39,000).

Table 6.5 Median weekly payment of occupational pension by social class, age, and sex (to the nearest £)

		Social Class						
		1 & 2		3n		3m		4 & 5	
		£	N	£	N	£	N	£	N
65–69	M	140	(69)	65	(96)	26	(141)	19	(94)
	F	132	(11)	40	(63)	19	(15)	19	(46)
70–74	M	130	(51)	29	(52)	26	(79)	21	(60)
	F	93	(9)	20	(40)	19	(12)	19	(44)
75–79	M	125	(35)	47	(23)	29	(48)	14	(26)
	F	103	(11)	50	(42)	11	(6)	19	(40)
80+	M	135	(12)	45	(20)	17	(38)	14	(20)
	F	48	(4)	20	(32)	19	(13)	19	(27)

Source: GHS, 1980.

A cohort effect on amount was present but not marked (Table 6.5). Women, except in Social Classes 4 and 5, and in Social Class 3 manual at age 80 and over, received smaller weekly pensions than men. The social-class differential overall was marked at all ages, particularly for men. In the 65–69 age-group, both men and women of professional and managerial classes had a median occupational pension seven times greater than that of those who had held unskilled or semi-skilled jobs. With the exception of older people from non-manual backgrounds, the amounts received in occupational pension were substantially less than the state pension. Consequently, for the majority of older people, occupational pensions provided a supplement to the basic state pension rather than a replacement for it.

Supplementary pension

This benefit was received by 18 per cent of the sample and the pattern of its receipt forms a mirror image of that for occupational pensions (Table 6.6). It increased with age, was higher amongst women than men and among the lower than the higher social classes. Thus, for households headed by women aged over 80 in Social Class 4 or 5, 42 per cent were receiving this pension. Given the problem of low take-up rates noted earlier this was almost certainly only a fraction of the proportion of older people actually entitled to receive this benefit.

Table 6.6 Percentages of elderly persons receiving supplementary pension by social class, age, and gender

| Social Class | Age | | | | | | | | | |
| | 65–69 | | 70–74 | | 75–79 | | 80+ | | All ages | |
	M	F	M	F	M	F	M	F	M	F
I & II	4	8	1	22	9	15	5	17	5	13
IIIn	6	9	4	12	16	14	18	20	8	12
IIIm	14	20	20	23	19	30	22	38	17	26
IV & V	17	21	23	30	29	37	24	42	22	30
All Classes	11	16	14	23	18	27	21	31	13	23
N	(699)	(810)	(507)	(613)	(298)	(477)	(195)	(368)	(1,698)	(2,268)

Source: GHS, 1980.

Pensioners formed the major client group of the SB system, although their pre-eminence has decreased since 1979. In 1948, 70 per cent of those receiving SB were pensioners compared with 57 per cent in 1984–5 (DHSS 1984). The decrease in the proportion of SB claimants who were pensioners should not be taken to imply an increase in living standards amongst elderly people; rather, it was the result of an increase in the number of long-term unemployed claiming this benefit.

There was very little difference between the median (£8.80) and mean (£9.83) payment or variation with age, sex or social class.

Unearned income

A substantial proportion of the sample, 41 per cent, reported that they had some unearned income. This proportion did not decrease significantly with age, nor was there a marked gender difference with the exception of households from Social Classes 4 or 5 (Table 6.7). The most striking variation was with social class: those from professional backgrounds were almost twice as likely to report unearned income of some kind than those from manual-occupation classes. That not all those from professional occupations reported some unearned income suggests that there may have been some under-reporting in response to this question.

Table 6.7 Percentages of older people receiving unearned income by social class and gender

Social Class	Male	Female	Total
1 or 11	64	63	63
111n	54	51	52
111m	49	46	48
IV or V	41	30	33
All classes	51	41	44
N	1,833	2,376	4,209

Source: GHS, 1980.

For the whole sample, the mean weekly value of unearned income was £5.09 and the median £1.19. The maximum amount of reported unearned income a week was £192.30p — an annual income of £9,999. Social class was the main influence on the median value of unearned income (Table 6.8). Households headed by men and women classified as belonging to professional groups had a substantially larger amount of unearned income than their counterparts in the manual groups. However, even for the former groups, this was substantially less than the amounts received in state and occupational pensions. Age did not seem to exert a marked influence upon the weekly amount received in unearned income. With the exception of Social Classes 1 and 2 there was little difference between men and women in the amounts received from this source.

Table 6.8 Median weekly unearned income by age, sex, and social class (to nearest £)

		Social Class			
		1 & 2 £ N	3n £ N	3m £ N	4 & 5 £ N
65–69	M	6 (91)	1 (95)	1 (138)	1 (81)
	F	2 (32)	1 (155)	1 (43)	1 (129)
70–74	M	5 (73)	1 (48)	1 (95)	0 (63)
	F	3 (28)	1 (101)	1 (36)	1 (100)
75–79	M	7 (43)	2 (27)	1 (62)	0 (34)
	F	2 (22)	2 (81)	1 (23)	1 (80)
80+	M	2 (23)	0 (19)	1 (39)	0 (24)
	F	4 (13)	1 (55)	1 (22)	0 (65)

Source: GHS, 1980.

Earned income

Of the 1980 GHS sample 5 per cent (227) reported that they had earnings from employment. This group consisted almost exclusively of men aged between 65 and 70 years of age and who were in Social Classes 1 or 2.

The prevalence of poverty

The prevalence of poverty amongst the 1980 GHS sample of older people was high. In 1980, 55 per cent of the elderly had an income within 140 per cent of the Supplementary Pension rate, the criterion which is now commonly used to define the poverty level (Townsend 1979). Using this definition the prevalence rose sharply with age, was always higher amongst women than men, and was most concentrated amongst those who had held manual jobs during their working lives (Table 6.9). Three main factors explain the distribution of poverty in later life — the level of the state retirement-pension; the heavy reliance of older people upon it and supplementary pension; and the non-availability of other sources of income.

The rate at which the state pension was paid would be of little importance if it had been a relatively unimportant source of income for older people. However, this was not the case. Almost three-fifths, 59 per cent, of the GHS sample in 1980 had no income other than that provided by the state, and for 75 per cent of them the retirement pension was their largest single source of income (Victor and Vetter 1986). Only for a minority did occupational pension payments exceed the amount they received in state pension.

The importance of the state as a source of income for older people

Table 6.9 The prevalence of poverty by age, sex, and social class

| | | Social Class | | | | | | | | |
| | | 1 & 2 | | 3n | | 3m | | 4 & 5 | | All classes | |
		N	%	N	%	N	%	N	%	N	%
65-69	M	(16)	12	(31)	22	(121)	44	(64)	36	(232)	31
	F	(13)	23	(193)	72	(59)	67	(276)	67	(541)	63
70-74	M	(31)	31	(34)	40	(98)	52	(77)	51	(240)	45
	F	(16)	41	(141)	73	(53)	78	(223)	73	(433)	71
75-79	M	(24)	34	(18)	40	(73)	62	(42)	59	(157)	51
	F	(19)	53	(104)	70	(48)	83	(181)	75	(352)	72
80+	M	(15)	43	(15)	42	(53)	66	(45)	69	(128)	59
	F	(12)	60	(80)	69	(48)	83	(148)	79	(288)	75
All ages	M	(86)	25	(98)	31	(345)	52	(228)	49	(757)	42
	F	(60)	39	(518)	71	(208)	76	(828)	72	(1,614)	70

Source: GHS, 1980.
'Poverty' = total individual income less than 140 per cent of the Supplementary Pension rate (£33.18p a week).

increased during the post-war period. In 1951, 42 per cent of pensioners' total income was derived from the state compared with 60 per cent in 1984-5 (DHSS 1984). Over the same period, earnings decreased in importance as an income source for older people. In 1951 they provided 27 per cent of total income and in 1984-5 only 9 per cent.

Conclusion

The analysis of the 1980 General Household Survey showed that the stereotypical views of older people as either poverty-stricken or affluent are inappropriate. There was a substantial range of income amongst older people and a complex relationship between age, gender, social class, and income. Overall, households headed by women, the very old, and those from the lower social classes were less well off than households whose heads were male, aged under 80 years who had held non-manual jobs. The variations in income levels reflect the differential access of older people to the main sources of income support in later life, especially to occupational pensions. Consistently, those households which had access to an occupational pension were substantially better off than those without such a pension. Thus, the distribution of income amongst older people very largely reflects the current effects of participation in the labour market before retirement. It is, therefore, reasonable to conclude that old age is not a leveller. As far as income is concerned, it represents the continuance and culmination of differentials established during working life.

Acknowledgements

I would like to thank the Office of Population Censuses and Surveys (OPCS), who carry out the General Household Survey, for allowing me to use the data, and also the ESRC data archive for preparing and distributing the data. The analysis was facilitated by the use of SIR files prepared at the University of Surrey by G.N. Gilbert, A. Dale, S. Arber and J. O'Byrne.

The 1980 GHS file used in the analysis was created by M. Evandrou.

My thanks also to the St. Mary's Hospital Special Trustees for financial support.

References

Beltram, G. (1984) *Testing the Safety Net*, Occasional Papers on Social Administration, No. 74, Bedford Square Press.

Bradshaw, J. (1985) 'Tried and found wanting: the take-up of means-tested benefits', in S. Ward (ed.) *DHSS in Crisis*, Child Poverty Action Group, pp. 102–11.

DHSS (1984) *Population, Pension Costs and Pensioners Incomes*, London: HMSO.

Fiegehen, G.C. (1986) 'Income after retirement', *Social Trends* (HMSO), pp. 13–18.

Groves, D. (1986) 'Occupational pensions', paper presented at the Annual Conference of the British Society of Gerontology, University of Glasgow.

OPCS (1986) 'General Household Survey 1985, Preliminary Results', *OPCS Monitor* GHS 86/1.

Phillipson, C. (1982) *Capitalism and the Construction of Old Age*, London: Macmillan.

Townsend,P. (1979) *Poverty in the United Kingdom*, Harmondsworth: Penguin.

Victor, C.R. and Evandrou, M. (1987) 'Does social class matter in later life?', in S.D. Gregorio (ed.) *Social Gerontology: New Directions*, London: Croom Helm.

Victor, C.R. and Vetter, N.J. (1986) 'Poverty, disability and use of services by the elderly', *Social Science and Medicine* 22 (10): 1087–91.

Walker, A. (1986) 'The politics of ageing in Britain' in C. Phillipson, M. Bernard, and P. Strang (eds) *Dependency and Interdependency in Old Age*, London: Croom Helm, pp. 30–45.

Chapter seven

Longitudinal Perspectives on the Living Arrangements of the Elderly

Emily Grundy

Introduction

At the start of the twentieth century those aged 65 and over represented
fewer than 5 per cent of the total population of England and Wales,
compared with over 15 per cent now. This change reflects the transition
from relatively high to low vital rates, most importantly the long-term
decline in fertility rates. The absolute size of the elderly population has
also increased considerably — by over 870,000 in the last quarter century
alone. This increase is the result of past falls in mortality at younger
ages, which resulted in increasing proportions surviving to old age, and
more recently has been influenced by falls in death rates among the elderly
themselves (Benjamin and Overton 1981; Grundy 1984). This latter
change has accelerated the rate at which the elderly population itself is
ageing. In the last decade (1976–86) the size of the whole elderly population aged 65 and over increased by less than 10 per cent, but the numbers
aged 85 and over went up by a third. In 1986 there were 639,000 very
old people aged 85 and over accounting for 1.3 per cent of the population as a whole; by the year 2006 those in this age group are projected
to number 1,116, 000 and constitute 2.1 per cent of the total population
(OPCS 1986).

These demographic changes are important because ageing is associated
with change in health status, socio-economic circumstances and family
and domestic situation. Morbidity and disability and the use of services
rise rapidly with age, particularly after the age of 80. Figure 7.1 shows
that National Health Service (NHS) expenditure on adults increases
steeply with age; and age variations in expenditure on personal social
services are even greater (VOPSS 1986). In a society with a long history
of collective support for elderly people (Smith 1984), the allocation of
resources to meet the needs of the increasing numbers of very old people
is an important policy issue.

Today's very old represent a selected group of survivors. It is known
that factors such as housing tenure and social-class membership are

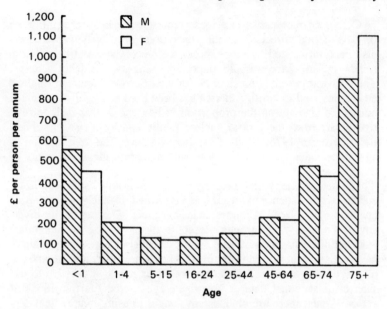

Figure 7.1 Per capita annual NHS expenditure by age and sex, Britain, 1983 (excluding maternity, administrative, and capital costs)

associated with the chance of survival both to and beyond the age of 65 (Palmore and Stone 1973; Fox *et al.* 1985), and also that the relationship between these and other variables and the risk of death may alter with age, partly because of the effect of selective survival. For example, smoking is a far less important risk factor for cardiovascular disease among the elderly than it is in middle age (Alderman and Stanback 1985).

Similarly, some of the characteristics of those who are currently old are cohort effects — that is to say, the outcome of specific and unique historical circumstances. Thus, 15 per cent of women aged 85 and over in 1981 were spinsters (compared with, for example, 5 per cent of 40–44 year-olds), reflecting the persistence into the early twentieth century of the historic European marriage pattern, which was characterized by high celibacy rates (Hajnal 1965), as well as a shortage of eligible men due to war and differential migration patterns when today's very old women were of marriageable age (Grundy 1983). In the same way, the relatively high proportion of very old people living in unfurnished privately rented accommodation is a legacy of the tenure patterns when they first set up home.

Cohort characteristics in a sense represent the long-term influence of past period effects: current generations of elderly people have also been influenced by more recent socio-economic and behavioural trends, including for example, important changes in residence patterns. The post-war period in much of North-west Europe, including England and Wales, and in North America has been marked by falls in average household size and in the proportion of households that include relatives apart from the central nuclear family and by a rise in solitary living (Kobrin 1976; Wall 1984; Burch 1985). The investigation of age-related changes in residence patterns forms the main focus of this chapter.

The heterogeneity of the elderly population is now well recognized, and an earlier tendency to regard it as a static and relatively homogeneous one has been replaced by interest in the dynamics of ageing and the diversity of the elderly age-groups. Recent analyses of cross-sectional data from national surveys, such as those presented elsewhere in this volume, have been helpful in demonstrating this heterogeneity; but while the use of appropriate statistical modelling techiques makes it possible to use such cross-sectional data to investigate age-related life transitions of various kinds, there are obvious advantages in using longitudinal data sets to do this.

This chapter presents some results of analyses of data from the OPCS Longitudinal Study (LS). The study is based on a 1 per cent sample of the 1971 Census population of England and Wales. Record linkage has been used to add to the data set details of routinely recorded demographic events, such as deaths, as well as information from the 1981 Census records of surviving sample members. The LS is a moving sample; members are lost through death and emigration and 1 per cent of births and immigrants are added in. This means that tables based on cross-sectional comparisons between 1971 and 1981 relate to separate but overlapping populations. Tables showing the 1981 characteristics of sample members include only survivors and, in the case of those aged 75 or more in 1971, only a minority of the original sample had survived.

Recent change in household size among the elderly

Table 7.1 shows the mean household size of LS sample members aged 60 and over in 1971 and 1981 in private (non-institutional) households. All the differences between 1971 and 1981 shown are statistically significant, except for the change in the small group of males aged 90 and over. The fall in mean household size reflects the trend towards greater residential independence among elderly people referred to earlier. In 1981, for example, 39 per cent of female and 20 per cent of male sample

Table 7.1 Mean household size among those aged 60 and over by age and sex, 1971 and 1981

Age	Males		Females	
	1971	*1981*	*1971*	*1981*
60–64	2.50	2.43	2.19	2.15
65–69	2.33	2.22	1.99	1.93
70–74	2.22	2.08	1.93	1.79
75–79	2.17	2.05	1.92	1.70
80–84	2.23	2.00	2.01	1.73
85–89	2.34	2.01	2.08	1.82
90 +	2.25	2.12	2.24	1.95
All 60 +	2.35	2.21	2.04	1.90

members aged 65 and over lived alone compared with 34 per cent and 13 per cent respectively ten years earlier. The proportions living outside a nuclear family but with other people (usually relatives), on the other hand, fell for women from 29 per cent to 14 per cent and for men from 13 per cent to 8 per cent (Grundy 1987a).

The higher mean household size of men compared with women in both 1971 and 1981 is chiefly a result of the much higher proportion married among the former. In 1981 only 8 per cent of women aged 85 or over were currently married, compared with 39 per cent of men. Figure 7.2 shows the marital status distribution of the elderly in 1981 by age and sex. Widows constitute half the female population at age 75, while widowers are a minority of the male population until the age of 87. Future generations of elderly people will include lower proportions of the never married (Timaeus 1986), but higher proportions of divorced people.

The age variations in mean household size reflect on the one hand declines in household size associated with the death and departure of co-residents and on the other, movement by some of the oldest into larger households with relatives. Household size thus falls with age until about the age of 80, as children still at home leave (15 per cent of men aged 65–69 in 1971, for example, were still living with their spouse and at least one never married child), and the proportion widowed increases.

The shift in household size as ageing takes place is best looked at longitudinally. Table 7.2 shows changes in household size between 1971 and 1981 for surviving sample members. Slightly over half the survivors were in the same size of household at both censuses. Among those not living alone in 1971, much larger proportions were living in smaller households ten years later than in larger ones. At the same time there

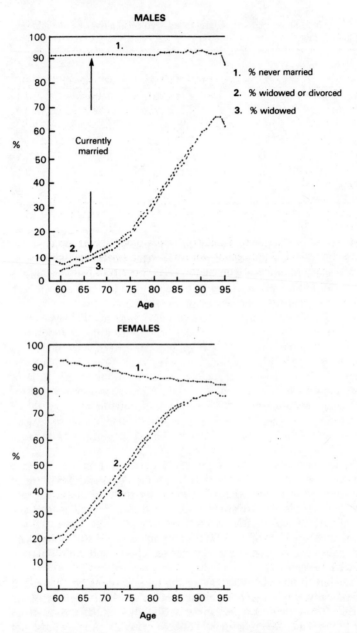

Figure 7.2 Men and women aged 60 and over by marital status and age, Britain, 1981

was an inverse relationship between household size in 1971 and the proportions resident in institutions in 1981: those living alone in 1971 were more likely to be in institutions ten years later than those in larger households.

There were also sex differences: some 10 per cent of women living alone in 1971 were in larger households in 1981, compared with 20 per cent of men. This difference partly reflects differences in remarriage: 8 per cent of 65–74 year-old men and 5 per cent of those aged 75 or over living alone in 1971 were in married couples ten years later, compared with only 1 per cent of 65–74 old women and as little as 0.1 per cent of women aged 75 or more (Grundy 1987a).

Changes in household size were also related to changes of address. Some 61 per cent of men and 63 per cent of women aged 65–74 living in a larger household in 1981 than in 1971 had moved, compared with only 32 per cent and 37 per cent respectively of those living in smaller households at the second date. Similarly, in the older age-group only 22 per cent of men and 32 per cent of women living in smaller households in 1981 had changed address, compared with 65 per cent of men and 55 per cent of women in larger households.

Changes in household size with age reflect life-cycle variations in co-residence patterns, and so involve changes in broad household type, as well as in household size. Figure 7.3 shows the proportion of survivors in the same broad type of household at both censuses by household type in 1971. The classification of family/household type is based on membership of a family — defined in strictly nuclear terms to include only lone parents with a co-resident, never married child and married couples with or without children and other co-residents — and relationship to household head. In a household containing a married couple and the wife's widowed sister, for example, the sister would be classified as living outside a family but with other people, while both spouses would be classified as living in a married-couple household.

It should be noted that the extent of change in the composition of elderly people's households is greater than shown in the figure, as residence in the same *type* of household does not necessarily mean co-residence with the same *people* or that there were no other changes in the inter-censal period. Over a third of those aged 75–84 in 1981 and nearly two-thirds of those aged 85 or over had lived in a different type of household ten years earlier. Change of household type between 1971 and 1981 was associated with change of address: over 40 per cent of those aged 65 and over in 1971 and still alive ten years later had moved; among those aged 75 or over in 1971 and still alive in 1981, a large proportion of the changes of address were accounted for by moves into institutions (Grundy 1987a).

Table 7.2 Changes in household size 1971–81 by household size in 1971 among those aged 65 and over in 1971

		1981 household size (%)									
	1971	Males					Females				
Age	Household size	Smaller	Same	Larger	NPH[a]	All	Smaller	Same	Larger	NPH[a]	All
65–74	1		72	20	8	100		81	10	9	100
	2	19	73	5	4	100	40	49	6	5	100
	3+	70	24	3	3	100	65	28	3	5	100
	All	29	61	6	4	100	31	56	7	6	100
75+	1		66	19	15	100		67	11	22	100
	2	25	56	8	11	100	31	41	11	17	100
	3+	52	35	1	12	100	52	33	3	13	100
	All	26	54	8	12	100	22	51	9	18	100

Note: a. NPH = Non-private household (institution)

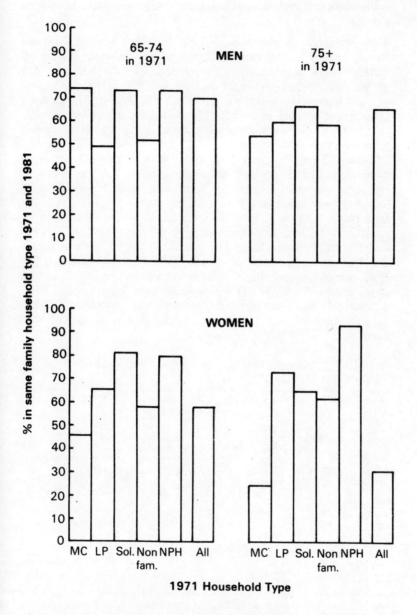

Figure 7.3 Percentage of men and women aged 65 or over in 1971 in the same broad family/household type 1971 and 1981, by family/household type in 1971

135

Socio-economic variations in household composition and household change

Socio-economic circumstances, and the interaction between them and the experience of events such as widowhood, may influence age-related variations in household size and composition. The mean household size of men aged 85–89 in 1981, for example, was 2.1 for those in owner-occupied housing, compared with 1.7 (SND = 5.34, P <0.001) for those in the privately rented sector. This difference partly reflects tenure variations in the composition of household types and partly transitions between different types of household.

Table 7.3 shows family and household type in 1981 for those living alone in 1971 by their tenure at the earlier date. In both age-groups a substantial majority of both sexes were still living alone in 1981; those who were local authority tenants in 1971 were the most likely to be still alone ten years later. Among those aged 75 and over quite large proportions were by 1981 in institutions or were lone parents or living outside a nuclear family but with others, generally relatives. The proportions who changed from living alone to living in this type of household (lone parent or with others) were highest among owner-occupiers and, except among older men, lowest among local authority tenants. Private tenants had the highest institutionalization rates. The data in the table also reflect the sex differential in remarriage referred to earlier.

Table 7.3 Family/household type in 1981 among those aged 65 and over and living alone in 1971, by 1971 tenure

Tenure in 1971		65–74					Age in 1971 *Family/household type in 1981 (%)*		75+			
		Soli-tary	Married couple	LP/ with others[a]	NPH[b]	N (=100%)	Soli-tary	Married couple	LP/ with others[a]	NPH[b]	N (=100%)
Owner	M	70	9	15	6	329	65	5	14	16	103
occupier	F	81	1	11	7	2,077	63	. .	16	21	625
Local											
authority	M	83	5	5	7	184	(75)	(7)	(9)	(9)	44
tenant	F	83	1	6	9	1,331	70	—	10	21	473
Private	M	68	8	11	13	205	(62)	(2)	(15)	(21)	48
renter	F	79	1	9	10	1,186	64	. .	12	23	414
All	M	73	8	11	8	721	67	5	13	15	195
	F	81	1	9	9	4,605	65	. .	13	21	1,512

Notes: a. LP/with others: Lone parent or living with others although not in a family.
    b. NPH: Non-private household (institution).
    . . < 0.5%
    ( ) denominator < 50

Table 7.4 shows those living in married-couple households in 1971 by their tenure then and their family and household type ten years later. Three-quarters of men aged 65–74 in 1971 and half of those aged 75 and over resident in such households in 1971 were in the same domestic situation in 1981; and the same was true of just under half the 65–74 year-old women but only a quarter of the older women, reflecting the different impact of widowhood on the two sexes. Owner-occupiers were the most likely to be still in married-couple households in 1981; the difference between owner-occupiers and local authority tenants was particularly marked among women aged 75 and over in 1971.

Table 7.4 Family/household type in 1981 among those aged 65 and over and living in married-couple households in 1971, by 1971 tenure

Tenure in 1971						Age in 1971				
			65–74					75+		
						Family/household type in 1981 (%)				
		Married couple	LP/ Soli-tary	with others[a]	NPH[b]	N (=100%)	Married couple	Soli-tary	LP/ with others[a]	NPH[b]	N (=100%)
Owner-	M	75	15	7	3	3,565	56	22	13	9	455
occupier	F	48	36	12	4	3,756	29	33	21	17	441
Local											
authority	M	72	17	7	4	1,406	52	29	11	8	137
tenant	F	44	39	12	5	1,649	18	45	16	20	194
Private	M	72	18	6	4	1,055	48	23	19	10	120
renter	F	41	40	14	5	1,277	23	39	22	16	158
All	M	74	16	7	3	6,030	54	23	14	9	713
	F	46	37	12	5	6,689	25	37	20	17	793

Notes: a. LP/with others: Lone parent or living with others although not in a family.
  b. NPH: Non-private household (institution).

Among those aged 65–74 and living in married-couple households in 1971, as among those living alone, tenants were slightly more likely than owner-occupiers to be in institutions by 1981. In the older age-group this was not always the case. However, if we take the entire sample aged 75 and over in 1971 and not just the married couples as we have done in Table 7.4, 11 per cent of male and 17 per cent of female owner-occupiers were in institutions in 1981 compared with 17 per cent and 20 per cent respectively of those in privately rented accommodation. Moreover, data analysed elsewhere show that tenure differentials in institutionalization persisted even after adjusting for the different age and marital-status composition of tenure groups (Grundy 1989).

Changes in household type between 1971 and 1981 were associated with both geographical movement and tenure change. Table 7.5 shows tenure continuity among women who had been in married-couple

Table 7.5 Percentage of women in married-couple households in 1971 living in same tenure in 1971 and 1981, by tenure in 1971 and family/household type in 1981

| 1971 | | | Family/household type in 1981 | | | | | |
Age	Tenure		Married couple	Lone parent	Solitary	With others	All in private households %	N
65–74	Owner-occupier		96	98	89	91	92	3,605
	Local authority tenant		93	90	94	61	91	1,566
	Private renter		59	48	59	36	56	1,216
	All in private	%	88	86	84	72	85	
	households	N	3,055	319	2,496	517		6,387
75+	Owner-occupier		84	(96)	88	93	92	368
	Local authority tenant		94	. .	99	14	89	156
	Private renter		50	. .	73	(14)	52	132
	All in private	%	87	(85)	88	65	83	
	households	N	201	39	293	123		656

( ) Denominator < 50
. . Denominator < 15

households in 1971 by family/household type in 1981. The 1971 tenants who by 1981 were living not in a family but with other people were much more likely to have changed tenure than were equivalent owner-occupiers, while tenure continuity among those living alone in 1981 was greatest among local authority tenants. This difference in tenure continuity partly reflects cohort differences in tenure: since there are higher proportions of owner-occupiers in younger age-groups, elderly people living in privately rented accommodation are less likely than elderly owner-occupiers to have younger relatives in the same tenure. There may also be variations in the ability of households in different sectors to provide accommodation for an elderly relative. As a result the tenure distribution of elderly people living in a household headed by a son or daughter in 1981 was very different from that of those living alone. Figure 7.4 illustrates this. It shows that a large majority of the women living with a son or daughter was in the owner-occupied sector and that this proportion varied little by age. Among those living alone, however, the proportion of owner-occupiers was much lower and lowest of all among the very old, a group which included the largest proportion of private renters.

Some of the tenure differences in change of household type between 1971 and 1981 may be the result of differentials in survival and widowhood. Figure 7.5 shows by tenure the proportions of men and women who were married in 1971 and still alive in 1981. Figure 7.6

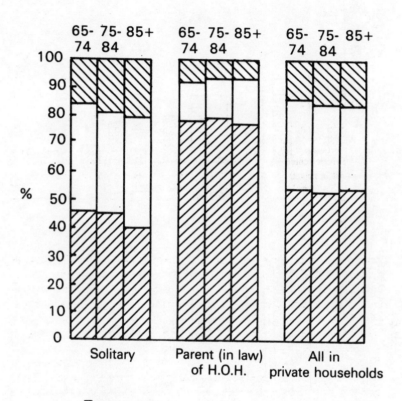

Figure 7.4 Elderly women living alone: as parent/parent-in-law of the head of household (HOH) and in all types of private household by tenure, (%) 1981

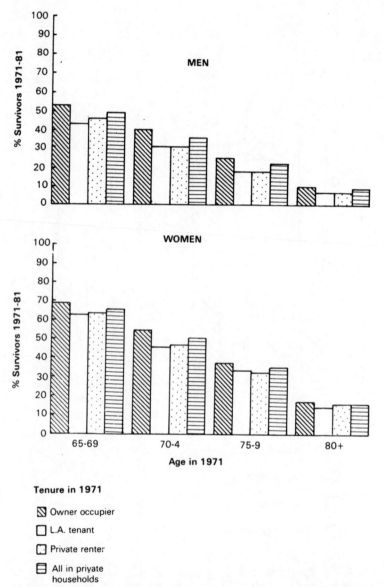

Figure 7.5 Survivors 1971–81 (%) among men and women aged 65 and over and married in 1971, by tenure in 1971

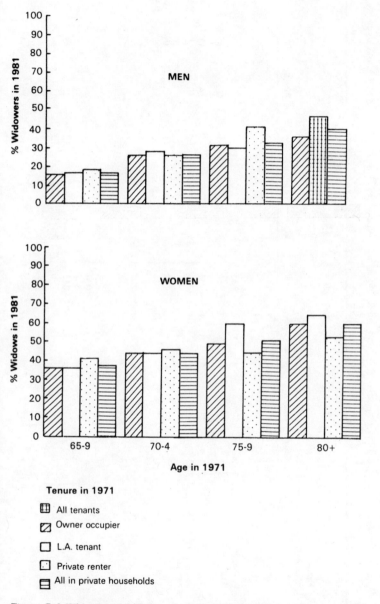

Figure 7.6 Widows and widowers in 1981 (%) among those who were married in 1971, by tenure in 1971

Table 7.6 Family/household type in 1981 by social class and family/household type in 1971 among men aged 65 and over in 1971

Social Class	1971 Family/household type	Age in 1971 Family/household type in 1981 (%)											
		65–74						75+					
		Married-couple	Solitary	LP/with others	Non-private	%	All N	Married-couple	Solitary	LP/with others	Non-private	%	All N
I & II	Solitary	7	72	15	6	9	138						
	MC	79	13	4	3	82	1,289						
	LP/with others	20	19	57	3	9	135						
	All[a]	67	19	10	3	100	1,577[b]						
III N	Solitary	10	71	11	6	11	103	4	62	14	14	17	71
	MC	78	13	6	3	81	789	55	19	17	10	66	272
	LP/with others	21	20	53	6	7	70[b]	4	12	71	13	16	68
	All[a]	66	20	11	3	100	974[b]	38	25	26	11	100	415[b]
III M	Solitary	9	79	6	6	10	204	5	67				
	MC	72	18	7	3	79	1,615	52	27				
	LP/with others	21	17	55	7	10	198[b]						
	All[a]	60	24	12	4	100	2,034[b]						
IV & V	Solitary	8	69	11	12	9	213	5	67	12	16	19	97
	MC	72	17	7	3	78	1,790	52	27	13	8	64	329
	LP/with others	19	17	57	7	12	265[b]	5	9	65	21	16	81[b]
	All[a]	60	22	13	5	100	2,294[b]	36	32	25	12	100	512[b]

Non-manual

Manual

| | | Age in 1971 Family/household type in 1981 (%) | | | | | | | | | | | |
| | | 65–74 | | | | | | 75+ | | | | | |
Social Class[d]	Family/household type 1971	Married-couple	Solitary	LP/with others	Non-private	%	All N	Married-couple	Solitary	LP/with others	Non-private	%	All N
Other[d]	Solitary	3	73	11	13	8	63	(4)[c]	(78)	(4)	(15)	14	27
	MC	71	16	9	4	72	547	58	22	10	10	58	112
	LP/with others	18	15	54	13	19	142	2	4	66	27	27	51
	All[a]	56	21	17	6	100	761[b]	35	25	25	15	100	192[b]
All	Solitary	8	73	11	8	9	721	5	67	15	15	17	195
	MC	74	16	7	3	79	6,030	54	23	14	9	64	713
	LP/with others	20	17	56	7	11	810	4	9	68	20	18	200
	All[a]	62	21	13	4	100	7,640[b]	36	28	24	12	100	1,119[b]

Notes: a. excluding those in non-private households in 1971.
b. including unclassified by family/household type.
c. ( ) denominator < 50.
d. including unclassified by social class.

shows the proportions among these survivors who by 1981 were widows or widowers, by tenure in 1971. Among men in all the age-groups over 65 in 1971, over half were dead by 1981; and those who were tenants in 1971 had a lower chance of survival than owner-occupiers. Larger proportions of women, particularly at younger ages, survived but tenure variations in survival were still apparent, although these diminished with age. The association between tenure and mortality has been shown elsewhere to weaken in older age-groups (Fox and Goldblatt 1982), probably both because of health-related movement from the rented sector to relatives' owner-occupied accommodation and because, particularly among men, those very old tenants still alive in 1981 represent a highly selected group of survivors with special characteristics.

Of those who did survive to 1981, owner-occupiers, as expected, tended to have lower widowhood rates than tenants (Figure 7.5). Sex differentials in mortality naturally influence the incidence of widowhood; because higher proportions of women than men survived to 1981, more of them were widowed in the inter-censal period.

In Table 7.6 household type in 1971 and 1981 is shown for men aged 65 or over in 1971 according to the Registrar General's Social Class classification. For retired men, allocation to social-class groups was made on the basis of stated pre-retirement occupation. The table suggests a positive association between 'higher' social class and living in a married-couple type household: such an association is the likely result of social-class variations in mortality and the incidence of widowhood. The 1971 household-type distribution of 1981 survivors, for example, shows that 82 per cent of men aged 65–74 in Social Classes I and II were in married couples compared with 79 per cent of those who had been skilled manual workers and 78 per cent of men in Social Classes IV and V. Men in non-manual social classes in this age-group in married couples in 1971 were also slightly more likely to be still in married couple households ten years later. Similar but less marked differences between the non-manual and manual categories are also apparent among those aged 75 or more in 1971. Both the proportion in married-couple-type households in 1971 and, of this, the proportion of survivors still in this type of household ten years later were lowest among men in the 'other and unclassified' social-class category. This group includes the permanently sick or disabled, as well as those not giving sufficient information at the time of the Census for assignment to a social-class category. Previous studies have shown that this group has particularly high mortality rates (Fox and Goldblatt 1982).

Table 7.6 also shows social-class variations in the proportions moving into institutions. In both age-groups the proportion in institutions in 1981 was highest for the 'other and unclassified' group and lowest for those in non-manual social-class groups. Among men aged 65–74 and living alone in 1971, those from Social Classes IV or V or in the unclassified group were twice as likely as other men to be in an institution ten years later. In the younger age-group, the proportion living in lone-parent households or non-family households with others in 1981 shows a 'U'-shaped distribution among those who had lived alone in 1971, being highest in the non-manual and the other-and-unclassified groups and lowest in Social Class III M. However, among men aged 75 or over in 1971, the proportion of those who had been living alone or in a married couple in 1971 and who in 1981 were lone parents or with others, was highest in the non-manual group.

The predominance of those from working-class backgrounds in institutions, which has been noted before (Townsend 1962), is undoubtedly related to their lower command of resources — including perhaps relatives able to provide accommodation — and poorer health status as indicated by social-class differentials in mortality (Fox *et al.* 1985) and reported morbidity (Grundy 1987c). It is also possiblethat the limited types of institutional care available may have particularly deterred those from non-manual backgrounds from seeking such accommodation. If this is so, the substantial growth in private residential homes which has occurred since 1981 (Grundy 1987b) may have influenced the relationship between social class and the probability of entering an institution. This will only be apparent if the data from this longitudinal study are further extended to include information from the 1991 Census, or if other data sources become available.

Conclusions

Socio-economic factors such as housing tenure and social class, it is clear, continue after the age of 65 to be associated with survival, widowhood, and transitions between different types of household. Tenants of both sexes and men in manual or unclassified social-class groups, for example, were more likely to enter institutions between 1971 and 1981 than owner-occupiers or men in non-manual occupations. Among those living alone in 1971, owner-occupiers and men in non-manual social-class groups were the most likely to be living in private households with relatives ten years later. However, both cohort and selection factors influenced the operation of these associations. Moving by tenants into the households of relatives, a transition which in itself may be related to health status, was often a move into the owner-occupied sector. This type of tenure transition would reduce the association between tenure and mortality risk in advanced old age.

Current trends in particular household and tenure arrangements, as well as age- and life-cycle-stage-related variations in marital and family status, also influence the household-type distribution of elderly people. Increases in the proportions living alone should not be taken to imply a greater tendency by younger relatives to abandon old people. Quite large minorities of the elderly, particularly women, lack close relatives (Abrams 1978), and those who do have families value residential independence. Thompson and West (1984), in a survey of residential preferences, found that moving in with relatives was an unpopular option for most. Elderly people who need help generally rely on relatives, whether or not they co-reside (Hunt 1978; Evandrou *et al.* 1986).

In short, the living arrangements of elderly people reflect their demographic and socio-economic history, their recent exposure to life-cycle events such as widowhood, age-related changes in health status, and their interaction with relatives and society as a whole — processes themselves influenced by socio-economic and behavioural change. Understanding the relationship between all these factors and age related changes in residence patterns, for example, is enhanced by the use of longitudinal data and the development of dynamic models of household and other transitions (Richards *et al.* 1987).

Acknowledgement

The author would like to thank all the OPCS staff concerned with the Longitudinal Study for their help.

References

Abrams, M. (1978) *Beyond Three Score Years and Ten: A First Report on a Survey of the Elderly*, Mitcham: Age Concern England.

Alderman, M.H. and Stanback, M.E. (1985) 'Hypertension', in A.N. Exton-Smith and M.E. Weksler (eds) *Practical Geriatric Medicine*, Edinburgh: Churchill Livingstone.

Benjamin, B. and Overton, E. (1981) 'Prospects for mortality decline in England and Wales', *Population Trends* 23: 22–7.

Burch, T. (1985) *Changing Age Sex Roles and Household Crowding: A Theoretical Note*, Proceedings of the XXth International Population Conference, Liège: IUSSP.

Evandrou, M. Arber, S., Dale, A., and Gilbert, G. (1986) 'Who cares for the elderly? Family care provision and receipt of statutory services', in C. Phillipson, M. Bernard, and P. Strang (eds) *Dependency and Interdependency in Old Age*, London: Croom Helm.

Fox, A.J. and Goldblatt, P.O. (1982) *Longitudinal Study: Socio-demographic Mortality Differentials*, London: HMSO.

Fox, A.J., Goldblatt, P.O., and Jones, D.R. (1985) 'Social class mortality differentials: artefact, selection or life circumstances?', *Journal of Epidemiology and Community Health* 39: 1–8.

Grundy, E. (1983) 'Demography and old age', *Journal of the American Geriatrics Society* 31: 325–32.

Grundy, E. (1984) 'Mortality and morbidity among the old', *British Medical Journal* 288: 663–4.

Grundy, E. (1987a) 'Household change and migration among the elderly in England and Wales', *Espace, Populations, Sociétés* 1: 109–23.

Grundy, E. (1987b) 'Community care for the elderly 1976–1984', *British Medical Journal* 294: 626–9.

Grundy, E. (1987c) 'Future patterns of morbidity among the elderly', in F.I. Caird and J. Grimley Evans (eds) *Advanced Geriatric Medicine 6*, Bristol: John Wright.

Grundy, E., (1989) 'Ageing: age related change in later life', in J. Hobcraft and M.J. Murphy (eds) *Population Research in Britain*, Oxford: Oxford University Press (in press).

Hajnal, J. (1965) 'European marriage patterns in perspective', in D.V. Glass and D.E.C. Eversley (eds) *Population in History*, London: Edward Arnold.

Hunt, A. (1978) *The Elderly at Home*, London: HMSO.

Kobrin, E.E. (1976) 'The fall of household size and the rise of the primary individual in the United States', *Demography* 13: 127–38.

OPCS (1986) *Population Projections, Mid 1985 Based*, OPCS Monitor PP2 86/1, London: OPCS.

Palmore, E. and Stone, V. (1973) 'Predictors of longevity: a follow up of the aged in Chapel Hill', *The Gerontologist* 13: 88–90.

Richards, T., White, M.J., and Tsui, A.O. (1987) 'Changing living arrangements: a hazard model of transitions among household types', *Demography* 24: 77–97.

Smith, R.M. (1984) 'The structured dependency of the elderly as a recent development: some sceptical historical thoughts', *Ageing and Society* 4: 409–28.

Thompson, C. and West, P. (1984) 'The public appeal of sheltered housing', *Ageing and Society* 4: 305–26.

Timaeus, I. (1986) 'Families and households of the elderly population: prospects for those approaching old age', *Ageing and Society* 6: 271–93.

Townsend, P. (1962) *The Last Refuge: A Survey of Residential Institutions and Homes for the Aged in England and Wales*, London: Routledge and Kegan Paul.

Voluntary Organizations Personal Social Services Group (VOPSS) (1986) 'The future of the social services: a discussion paper', London: VOPSS (c/o MIND).

Wall, R. (1984) 'Residential isolation of the elderly: a comparison over time', *Ageing and Society* 4: 483–503.

Part III

Contemporary Studies of Old People and their Carers

Chapter eight

Virtue and Vicissitude:
The Role of Old People's Clubs†

Dorothy Jerrome

Introduction

The research described here had several objectives. An earlier study of middle-class friendships in later life had thrown up a number of questions. One concerned class and gender differences in the pattern and significance of intimate relationships in later life, another social processes in the elderly peer group, and, at a more general level, the experience of ageing among peers and in age-mixed settings. An extensive American literature exists on all these questions, but very little work has taken place in Britain on any of them. Some of the American literature and its possible application to British society has been summarized elsewhere (Jerrome 1982, 1985).

This chapter presents the findings of a recent British study of peer-group processes in old age. It begins with a brief account of the research from which the analysis is derived. There follows a description of activities in old people's clubs and an analysis of the symbolic significance of words and actions. Discussion turns to the personal and social consequences of participation in peer-group rituals. Attitudes to ageing in the elderly peer group and collective responses to it are seen to provide normative guidelines for individual old people encountering the vicissitudes of age. Analysed in detail, the behaviour of elderly association members indicates a particular model of ageing. Conformity to it is rewarded by a sense of virtue and by status within the peer group; but not everyone has access to the leadership roles which allow incumbents to demonstrate their worthiness. The operation of the model of ageing dominant in club culture is linked to the fate of the organizations themselves. The discussion ends with a brief account of change and continuity in old age organizations.

---

† This chapter is a shortened version of a longer paper. The full version of which can be obtained from the author on request.

The Role of Old People's Clubs

Background

In January, 1985, I started an anthropological research project in Brighton. My methods were intensive, involving mainly participant-observation and unstructured interviewing. I was involved with nine old people's clubs and a church community, which included a number of age-graded organizations. Over the eight months of field-work and a further ten months of sporadic contact with members, I attended about forty club meetings and went on three outings. I attended a great many business, devotional, and social meetings in the church. I got to know approximately 170 people, ranging in age from late thirties, to mid-nineties, but most were in their seventies and eighties. I have detailed information on fifty-five of them.

As is the nature of anthropological research, the focus of attention shifted as fieldwork progressed. New issues emerged as highly significant in the ageing experience of my informants. A detailed analysis of my material drew my attention in particular to the role of ritual in the social construction of old age.

Peer group rituals

It is suggested in the literature that social status is one of a number of areas of ambiguity in retirement. On departure from the work-force the basis of social assessment shifts from achievement to ascription. Previous identities become meaningless. Cultural prescriptions are vague or lacking (Rosow 1967). Myerhoff (1984) talks about the difficulty of discontinuity in cultural conditioning. There occurs a reversal of expectations from active and assertive to passive and serene. In the anthropological literature, elderly people are seen as being in a state of liminality: in limbo between the fixed and regulated stages of mid-life and extreme old age (Keith 1982; Myerhoff 1984). Like adolescents, they are on the threshold of a new experience.

Although undefined, old age has negative associations. The emphasis on individualism and self-reliance in our society reduces the status of older people who, in the absence of paid employment or other social contributions, are seen as having nothing of cultural value to trade with the young in return for support. Their relations with the young are, therefore, non-reciprocal and hence tainted with dependency (Clark 1969). In such circumstances, the peer group assumes significance (Dono et al. 1979; Harris 1983). Members of a single cohort, with common expectations based on a shared past, are a source of moral and practical support (Jerrome 1985).

One of the most important functions of the peer grouping is to engage in collective rituals which dramatize and ameliorate their situation

(Hockey 1983; Myerhoff 1984). For ritual — in the sense of a series of patterned acts having symbolic significance, a significance related to the wider social situation of the participants — is prominent in all areas of uncertainty, anxiety, impotence, and disorder. By its repetitive character it provides a message of pattern and predictability. There are some groups of elderly people in particular whose social invisibility calls for symbolic and ritual elaboration. The circumstances of elderly ethnic minorities, of groups who have lost their natural progeny to carry on their stories and traditions, and of people without natural heirs and witnesses to validate their claims to have led worthy lives, generate ritual in old age. Faced with the erosion of traditional values (authority, patriotism, duty, family life) in contemporary Britain they seek constantly to affirm their belief in such values through symbolic display.

The weekly meetings of club and fellowship, which I observed, can be seen as what Myerhoff (1984: 320) calls 'definitional ceremonies', ritualized performances that 'provide arenas for garnering honour and prestige, for enacting and displaying one's own interpretation of oneself, against the play of accident, chaos and negative interpretations that may be offered up by history and outsiders.

Old people's clubs

The weekly meetings of both club and fellowship follow a set pattern which goes on unchanged year after year. The pensioners' clubs invariably start with singing, of either a hymn or the club song, and this is followed by a prayer. Then comes the business part including apologies for absence, the minutes of the previous meeting, matters arising, and brief reports from the secretary, treasurer, and social secretary, the latter dealing with forthcoming outings, holidays, and other social events. Next, with slight variations, comes the birthday song, with the distribution of a card, a hug, and a small gift of soap or chocolate to every one who has had a birthday in the previous week. Extra applause is merited by the achievement of a great age especially in the event of recent ill health or other adversity. The sick news, which follows, brings members up to date on the condition of people absent through ill health. Returning members are welcomed back to seats which will have been kept for them, sometimes for many months, and applauded for their effort.

The business, which tends to last about twenty minutes, is concluded with refreshments. The consumption of a cup of tea and two biscuits, and the lively conversation which accompanies it, is an important part of the meeting (in the view of the organizers).

The second half of the meeting is given to 'the entertainment', in those clubs not devoted to weekly bingo sessions, typically taking the form of a presentation by a visiting concert party of songs, sketches, jokes, readings, and instrumental items with as much audience participation as possible; or members themselves organizing quizzes, sing-a-longs, items for solo voice, piano recitals, readings, and recitations. Members join in the choruses or sing along with the soloist throughout, often word perfect. The rendering of Land of Hope and Glory and other patriotic songs, Old Father Thames, Sussex-by-the-Sea, and so ↵ are responded to with warmth and vigour. Occasionally there is dancing and, periodically, a party to mark religious festivals (Easter, Christmas) or the anniversaries of important national events such as VE Day and the Queen's Coronation. The final item is a raffle of groceries, flowers, and other small items contributed by members to raise funds for the club. The meeting ends with the club song or hymn such as 'God be with you 'til we meet again'. This is sometimes followed by auld lang syne, hands linked where seating permits.

Many of these activities have symbolic significance. Thus the shared reading of the Lord's prayer, gabbled off in the upstairs room of a pub as a prelude to the real business of the afternoon, can be understood not so much as a religious ritual but as a symbol of unity and continuity and of the members' location in time, survivors of an age when religious belief and organized religion were more significant. Other activities, from the informal rituals of greeting and parting and tea drinking, to the formal applauding, singing, and collective reminiscing, underline values and express important allegiances — to the age group, to the moral community of the club, to friends, and to members of one's personal network. Throughout, the meeting is punctuated by recurrent themes: the importance of friendship and caring, of self-help and struggle, of patriotism and family life. Some expressions are repeated week after week, year after year: 'Thank you for all the gifts on the table, and for any help you give the club in any way', 'Now let us end in the usual way.'

The recurrent themes and phrases, the prescribed responses, and modes of participation provide security, a sense of personal location in time, a link between the individual and the collective. The intensity of emotional involvement, particularly apparent during the ritual singing and entertainment, heightens feelings of solidarity and gives sensory experience of continuing existence and vitality.

Association with peers — formal and informal — brings with it a range of benefits: an opportunity for self-expression, a sense of security, a supportive network, a chance to confront some of the ambiguities and losses of ageing. The literature on social support confirms the influence of peers and significant others in the perception of one's condition and control of the emotional consequences (Craney 1985). A cultural rather than a psychological perspective alerts us to the possibility that the incessant talk about anything which is a source of problems and uncertainties is part of a process of social construction. Good health is rarely discussed. Indeed, it is often made light of. On the other hand, ill health and responses to it, housing problems, any topic involving moral judgements and hence relevant for the creation of norms, is debated at length. Such a view of reality as socially constructed has much in common with Vesperi's (1985) analysis of ageing in Florida. In the 'city of green benches', individual actors are guided by messages about age, coming from the social milieu of friends, neighbours, relatives, fellow club-members, and service providers. For it is 'in the interstices of daily living, in the commonplaces of conversation and the "informal formalities" of social interaction, that the cultural construction of old age unfolds' (ibid.: 48). Members of the social network are vital in contributing to the formation of attitudes. It is largely through informal exchanges that private experiences are transformed into shared public knowledge and attributed with meaning.

A context for ageing

Viewed as a context for ageing, the peer group is seen to confer signifi-cant advantages on its members. Together, members work out appropriate ways of behaving in what is, in some senses, a normative vacuum. Individual responses to ill health, bereavement, and other age-related problems are compared and assessed in terms of collective standards. Models of successful ageing are reflected in the ritual celebration of birthdays.

Assumptions about successful ageing are also contained in the detailed and lengthy sick news, the welcome extended to members returning after illness, and the approval bestowed on the widow or widower who copes well with bereavement. Members are socialized to new roles and given a chance to get used to them in a supportive setting, and some, like Michael who was forced to find an alternative to his earlier self-image of a successful professional man, actively seek confirmation of their new identities.

The virtue of coping is expressed in conversation, in song and in exhortation from the platform. It is supported by passages from Francis Gay's books, the main source of public readings, and a popular gift for private consumption. *The Friendship Book*, by Francis Gay, is published annually. It contains a reading for every day of the year, and its texts, jokes, and moral homilies offer guidance on how to evaluate experience. In particular, it indicates ways of dealing with adversity: struggle and stoicism on the one hand and resignation and acceptance on the other. 'Count your blessings' and 'Every cloud has a silver lining' are import-ant principles. Visiting entertainers, club leaders, and individual members of old people's clubs, and in the Christian fellowships the speakers, leaders, and members, all choose passages from current and earlier

Friendship Books along these lines — passages illustrating the value of coping, the importance of being happy, and the link between the two: being reconciled to one's lot brings quiet satisfaction and spiritual strength. It also makes one easier to live with, and so reduces the burden one's frailty might impose on other people.

In the culture of the clubs there is a close association between ill health and self-definitions of 'old', a phenomenon widely noted in the literature (Stephens 1976; Williams 1986). You are old when ill health produces a change in life-style. In the sick news, shifts in age status occur as individuals are deemed to have moved, through chronic ill health, into a new category. When Mrs J, an active church worker in her eighties, talks of visiting old people, she refers to their health status rather than their chronological age. Responses to both ill health and old age are similar: struggle and resistance are seen as possible and desirable. Surrender without struggle is a sign of moral weakness. Attendance at meetings is visible proof of struggle and hence of virtue. Social participation entails an expression of a notion of ageing well.

Death in a religious setting

Death marks the end of direct involvement in the club but indirect involvement continues, sometimes for months. Death, a regular occurrence, is treated quite differently in club culture compared with the community at large, where it is hardly treated at all. The peer group compensates for what Elias (1985) and others have noted as a general reluctance to acknowledge death. In the club, the elderly member confronts death in a supportive setting. The implication for the living of the rituals surrounding death, of the frequent talk about a deceased member, their manner of dying, their possible whereabouts, their loss to the community, is that death is a part of life, not outside it. A life is put in context; there is continuity between past and future. Above all, death is normal: 'Death? — that's life!' — and so members are prepared for loss and their own eventual deaths.

In the religious organizations the pattern of ritual acknowledgement of death is slightly different, with explicit references to continuity of existence, 'eternal life', and continued membership of the collectivity, 'the communion of saints'. In other respects, too, the fellowships provide a different context for ageing, integrated as they are into an age-mixed church community.

The models of ageing held out to elderly people in the church, while similar to those of the club in terms of their central values, are set in the context of a church career with clearly defined stages. The stages in the typical career vary according to gender and age. With slight variations, the career path of older men and women has started with membership of the Sunday School and the Boys' or Girls' Brigade — the gateway to church membership, administration, and junior leadership roles — or the youth club, another gateway to adult church roles or entry via courtship and marriage. This is followed by Sunday School teaching, highly esteemed and publicly acclaimed work, and membership of church organizations. Minor church work and more demanding involvement through stewardship and membership of church committees follows. From this the older man retires to become an elder statesman. His wife, who has taken on only a limited amount of committee work, is likely to be involved still in sick visiting and women's organizations. The final stage follows death when one is remembered in prayer, legacy, and legend. Movement from one stage to the next is justified not simply in terms of the individual's needs and capacities but with reference to the instrumental and expressive orientation of the group.

Notions of service and struggle occur as part of the Vision (of God's Kingdom on earth) which unites believers of all ages. Membership of a close-knit age-mixed organization provides a distinctive experience of ageing, social change, and replacement. The reciprocal expectations of people at different points in the church career create an effective system of socialization and social control. Conformity to age roles is underpinned by the network and legitimated by Christian values. The old person in the church enjoys the security of a highly integrated and purposeful existence.

Models of ageing

Ideas about ageing well and ageing badly abound in the elderly peer group and outside it. On close inspection of the club population it appears that, while the chronological age range is substantial, (members range from early sixties to early nineties), the crucial dimensions of differentiation are social age and attitudes to ageing. Age enters people's calculations in a number of ways. It is frequently used as an excuse for giving up responsibility, at any age from 60 onwards; and it is used as a socially acceptable excuse in place of what may be the real reasons for giving up: boredom, lack of interest, changing priorities. The use of age to discontinue former practices occurs at the organizational level, too. People are said to be too old to parade around in Easter bonnets, an explanation which conveniently overlooks the less flattering facts: a misunderstanding last year between the secretary and the adjudicator, the ill-grace of the losers and their friends, and so on.

The same sort of rationalization goes on in the case of people who use age to avoid taking on office. In most cases the people concerned have never held office but now they use age to justify their position. Age is used widely to defend one's activities as part of a personal strategy to conserve energy. At the same time, age is used by younger people as a basis for allocating jobs to their elders. On the assumption that older people need an occupation, have plenty of spare time, and are not the best judges of their own capabilities, retired unattached men and women are mercilessly pounced upon by younger people — organizers of voluntary agencies, church workers — who have work to be done. To outsiders it might seem that the elderly incumbents are hanging on to office. In reality it is often made impossible for them to retire. The pressure upon them to remain in office is backed up by an ethic of service to the community, the need for a purposeful existence, the importance of activity, doing rather than being (especially in old age), and other cultural values.

The different and contradictory ways in which age is used reflect the cultural vagueness surrounding this dimension of experience. While on the one hand, cultural freedom and confusion produce the need for ritual elaboration, they also provide scope for manipulation and the promotion of personal interests. They provide calculating, resourceful elders with a set of possibilities for innovation, and for the exploitation of the rolelessness which characterizes retirement (Rosow 1967; Myerhoff 1984).

The notion of individual freedom and scope for manoeuvre, however, must not be taken too far. Social situations cannot be defined unilaterally. They have to be negotiated (albeit on one person's terms). Individual freedom is limited by other people who can withhold confirmation of the subjective account. The need for the social legitimation of self-definitions of old age is similar to that required for subjective experiences of ill-health noted earlier. Health and illness are not clearly differentiated aspects of reality. Illness is defined in terms of inactivity, so the existence of social roles and relationships from which to withdraw is crucial for knowledge of one's condition (Herzlich 1973). Similarly, personal constructions of old age are dependent on confirmation by others. This principle — the intersubjectivity of experience in old age — is clearly at work in the church community.

Ageing in the church

Officially, age is not an organizing principle or criterion for distinction in the church, though unofficially, popular stereotypes and theories of ageing abound. An ideology of family and fellowship unites people across the generations. Distinctions are made on the basis of adherence to these shared values, and perfection in the performance of Christian duty.

Age is no barrier to participation in The Work. The activity principle is applied by the young most vigorously to older people whose involvement is functional: if, in response to pressure, they hang on in spite of personal misgivings, they are held in high regard. They are treated with deference by those at the commanding heights of church organization (in their fifties and sixties). They become folk heroes and heroines, even legends in their time. Patterns of deference reveal these old people as repositories of cultural values (Maxwell 1986). The cultural vagueness influencing individual strategies may thus be observed at an organizational level too. In the absence of clear rules for transition into and out of positions of responsibility, pressure is applied to the elders to produce conformity to a model which is functional for the organization. The result is a pattern which does not always accord with individual capacity, as in the case of Mr Stubbs who, in his mid-seventies and suffering from arthritis, was anxious to cut down on his church commitments but had his protests brushed aside.

The cultural context

Concepts of old age in church and club, like those of ill health, need to be understood in their cultural context. A complex of values, such as autonomy and achievement, and popular notions of ageing, such as the importance of activity and social involvement, combine to influence the models of ageing which provide the basis for personal strategies and the evaluation of other people's performance. The relationship between these sets of influences can be presented diagrammatically, as is illustrated in Figure 8.1.

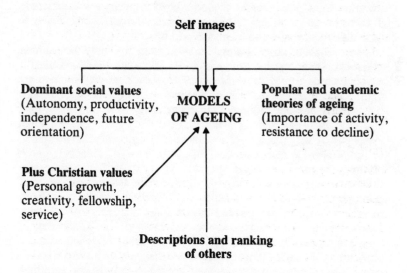

Figure 8.1 Influences on models of ageing

According to the model of old age dominant among club members and church-goers, to be really old is to be functionally impaired. Old age should be resisted, though surrender is legitimate after a struggle. People are ranked in terms of their approximation to the ideal. The 'wonderful' person is an achiever who performs well in the face of adversity. His or her qualities of intelligence, judgement, and stoicism inspire admiration and respect. The 'great' person is all these things and a model of Christian or community service too. Both the wonderful and the great are remembered after their time. The merely 'lovely' are not, though their beautiful characters inspire feelings of warmth and affection. The 'poor thing' by contrast is a pitiful creature unable to cope with adversity. Old age is thus a moral category. Responses to it are a matter of virtue and moral strength or weakness. To be happy and make the best of things in spite of pain or hardship is a moral and social obligation attached to the status of old or handicapped or unattached persons in our society.

Virtue and vicissitude

The resistance model of ageing provides an explanation for failure and unhappiness in the principle of just deserts: 'You get out of life what you put into it.' It also offers a standard against which to evaluate one's performance. Some old people do this much more openly than others: remarks like 'I am always happy, I set an example to others' and 'I fill my time doing good works' suggest a need to justify one's existence. They betray an uncertainty and insecurity arising from the changing basis of self-evaluation in retirement and widowhood.

Most people do not proclaim their virtue quite so openly. Strong identities and coping mechanisms perfected over a life time help them to accept their decline in status (Streib 1976). However, they still respond to the loss of status by making a career out of ageing. Old people acquire a sense of achievement from the accomplishment of small routines. Each day is a challenge and its conquest essentially a competitive affair (Stephens 1976). Over the years the routines may become private rituals to compensate, at least partially, for the absence of public ceremonial marking the progression through old age.

The success ethos of modern western society is thus adapted to the conditions of old age. For middle-class elderly the values of achievement and independence are sustained through the pursuit of a middle-aged life-style. The effects of illness and status loss are minimized and ageing is denied (Clark 1969; Hellebrandt 1980) or tolerated as an opportunity for personal development (Williams, 1986). Working-class elderly people vary in their responses: according to Williams, surrender is more typical than resistance. In the club population, however, the values of achievement and independence remain sacrosanct.

Regardless of social background, health and fitness appear to be crucial for the sense of ageing. In the club population attitudes are ambivalent. Illness creates a dilemma resolved by a compromise between the ideal of resistance and the less-valued response of surrender. Diminishing resources are sometimes protected by a strategy of change: a cutting down, a giving up in one area is balanced by an intensification of interest in another, less strenuous kind of activity. The exchange of roles between secretary and chairman as the former becomes increasingly frail, or the move from secretary to treasurer, is carefully presented as a 'slowing down' rather than a 'giving up'.

For people with multiple or severe handicaps, accommodating to disability becomes a governing principle. Life is lived within strictly defined limits imposed by ill health. However, with almost all the club populations, health issues loom large in thought, conversation, and ritual. The general interest in health might, as Stephens suggests in relation to inner-city hotel residents (1976), rest on a fear of one's own loss of freedom and valued life-style. In the culture of the club and fellowship, health issues form part of the dialogue through which norms of illness behaviour in old age are negotiated (Jerrome 1986). Whichever the case, the presence of witnesses and fellow sufferers is essential for knowledge of one's own condition.

People in old people's clubs and fellowships tend to be natural resisters: that is why they are there. Social participation is part of a strategy for survival. All are determined to keep going, either by denying illness or acknowledging it and coming to terms with it. The latter course — acknowledgement and compromise — is sometimes adopted reluctantly in response to pressure from friends and relatives. These others become involved when denial that anything is amiss threatens to make the condition worse.

Virtue: a limited resource

Nevertheless, the battle against old age is generally waged independently of and if necessary at the expense of peers. Despite the rhetoric of friendship and solidarity a gulf exists between the relatively active members in the club or fellowship and the relatively passive. In their different styles of participation the first compete with the second to age well. The most active — leaders and committee members — make distinctions between themselves and the rest, who are said to be lonely, passive, demanding, sometimes suspicious and ungrateful, and often childlike. The relatively passive members in turn are critical of the organizers and resentful of their privileges. They often regard club officials, the latter's friends, and people with leadership pretensions with suspicion. They are particularly critical of those who operate without any checks on their behaviour by a committee. This is not to deny the widespread warmth and mutual respect between many leaders and club members. At all times, however, a sense of 'us' and 'them' pervades meetings, matched by social and physical boundaries which separate the leaders and active members from the rest.

The preservation of the status quo allows the active workers to regard themselves as an élite in physical, and hence in moral, terms. They find confirmation of their superiority in their public achievements. Their unusual energy and ability to cope with sometimes severe health problems are reaffirmed. In these circumstances, it becomes increasingly difficult to give up. Surrendering office is to surrender control over the ageing process. To the extent that club work is a joint project shared by a married couple or group of friends, giving it up would also have implications for one's social network.

The ageing of associations

The significance of office to those who hold it might account for an interesting feature of old age organizations: the tendency of clubs and fellowships to age and die with their leaders. A decline in numbers in the clubs I studied and in others for which I have information seems to be related to the age of the founders and their inability to match losses through death or disability with new recruits. The same is true of the church-based groupings I studied. The life cycle of the organization appears to match that of its founder members, who carry it forward with them. Rather than belonging to the age grade, with long-term members passing out at one end and new members moving up from the grade below, the club becomes the property of a particular age set. The tendency for voluntary bodies — particularly, expressive associations where the quality of personal interaction is expected to be a major source of gratification — to be age-graded, is quite common, even when they are officially open to anyone regardless of age (Fennell 1981; Unruh 1983). What is interesting is the strength of identification of the clubs and fellowships with a quite specific age cohort. There are various possible explanations for this. One such is the unattractiveness of club culture for cohorts now reaching retirement age. The unique historical experiences which turned the present cohorts of club members into a generation, with all that that implies for identity and outlook have less meaning for them. (Jerrome 1988). I would argue, however, that the explanation lies less in generational differences than in social age and attitudes to ageing.

Club rituals are, it is true, expressions of generational distinctiveness. They also express ideas about the ageing process. Participation, I have argued here, can be viewed as a personal strategy for demonstrating fitness and the capacity for survival. While both members and leaders are distinguished from non-members by their choice of this form of social activity, participation in club life assumes special significance for the leadership. An analysis of power and authority in old age organizations indicates personal strategies for ageing which make retirement from office difficult. Thus, the club or fellowship ages with its executive committee and ultimately expires.

In traditional age-set societies, where age is the organizing principle and the age-set the basic social unit, the movement into and out of office is a societal problem, managed collectively. In our society the timing of transitions is more an individual than an age-set problem, though response to the problem is sometimes made collectively. The National Federation of Retirement Pensioners' Associations has tried to halt the decline of the movement by introducing compulsory retirement from office at 80. This, it is thought, would defeat the problem of elderly married couples who not only hang on to senior posts but expel their opponents. Proposals to this effect have so far been outvoted by the over 80 year-olds on the national executive committee. It has also been suggested that elderly leaders appoint younger deputies, but that would undermine the traditional basis of nomination and recruitment to office.

The Methodist Church's governing body recently introduced a six-year rule to prevent elderly incumbents from hanging on to office. Church offices may be held for six years only, and two years must elapse before renomination. Informal responses to the problem of age transitions include secessions by the younger element and occasional coups by factions in clubs.

Conclusion

Like other writers on the subject of peer grouping in later life, I see old age organizations as a response to the special nature of the retirement phase, with its ambiguities of status and role. The shift in the basis of social assessment and the absence of clearly defined social roles makes this a difficult time in which members of the peer group have a valued role as providers of moral and practical support. Ritual behaviour is important at times of doubt and uncertainty. In this phase the peer group engages in collective rituals which both express and ameliorate the situation of normlessness and cultural confusion. Club and fellowship meetings are vehicles through which elderly members affirm their belief in tradition, their solidarity with one another, and their adherence to shared standards of behaviour.

Members of old age organizations enjoy a range of benefits. Membership provides an opportunity for self-expression, a sense of security, a supportive network, and a chance to confront some of the losses and ambiguities of ageing with others undergoing the same experience. These losses include previous statuses and identities, important relationships, health and life itself. The club provides a context for socialization to new roles. Together, members establish through conversation and formal utterance, through song, prayer, music and various kinds of ritual performance, new ways of behaving in what would otherwise be essentially a normative vacuum. Club and fellowship members share a model of ageing which stresses struggle and resistance, a model which needs to be understood in its cultural context. Cultural vagueness gives scope for manipulation, permitting age to be used in a variety of ways to promote personal interests. At the same time, a cultural emphasis on activity, achievement, and self-reliance, combined with notions of service and fellowship, influence personal strategies. Old age organizations are arenas for the acquisition of virtue, since social participation is proof of the ability to cope with the vicissitudes of age. However, as participation is a strategy for survival, and a sign of moral strength, so withdrawal amounts to moral weakness. Since there is a limit to the number of leadership roles, the pursuit of virtue is a competitive process. Retirement from office is particularly difficult, for leadership roles are a sign of activity par excellence. However, the decision to go is a personal one, for in our society the timing of age transitions is largely an individual matter, not one which is handled collectively. In these circumstances the incumbents hang on to office and the clubs expire with them. The attainment of virtue is in the end at the clubs' expense.

Acknowledgement

The study on which this chapter is based was funded by the ESRC, Grant No. 1250005.

References

Clark, M. (1969) 'Cultural values and dependency in later life', in R. Kalish (ed.) *The Dependence of Old People*, Ann Arbor: University of Michigan Press.
Craney, M. (1985) 'Interpersonal support and health of older people', in W. Peterson and J. Quadagno (eds) *Social Bonds in Later Life*, California: Sage.
Dono, J., Falke, C., Kail, B., Litwak, E., Sherman, R., and Siegel, D. (1979) 'Primary groups in old age', *Research on Ageing* 1(4): 403–43.
Elias, N. (1985) *The Loneliness of the Dying*, Oxford: Blackwell.
Fennell, V.I. (1981) 'Friendship and kinship in older women's organisations', in C. Fry *et al. Dimensions: Ageing, Culture and Health*, New York: J.F. Bergin.
Gay, F. (1985) *The Friendship Book of Francis Gay*, London: D.C. Thomson & Co.
Harris, C.C. (1983) 'Associational participation in old age', in D. Jerrome (ed.)

Ageing in Modern Society, London: Croom Helm.

Hellebrandt, F.A. (1980) 'Ageing among the advantaged', *Gerontologist* 20(4): 404–17.

Herzlich, C. (1973) *Health and Illness*, London: Academic Press.

Hockey, J. (1983) ' "Just a song at twilight", residents' coping strategies expressed in ritual form', in D. Jerrome (ed.) *Ageing in Modern Society*, London: Croom Helm.

Jerrome, D.M. (1982) 'The significance of friendship for women in later life', *Ageing in Society* 1(2).

Jerrome, D.M. (1985) 'Voluntary association and the social construction of old age', in A. Butler (ed.) *Ageing* London: Croom Helm.

Jerrome, D.M. (1986) 'Me Derby, you Joan', in C. Phillipson (ed.) *Dependence and Independence in Old Age*, London: Croom Helm.

Jerrome, D.M. (1988) 'That's what it's all about: old people's organisations as a context for ageing', *Journal of Ageing Studies* 2(1): 71–81.

Johnson, F., & Aries, E. (1983) 'The talk of women friends', *Women's Stud. International Forum* 6(4): 353–61.

Keith, J. (1982) *Old People as People* Toronto: Little, Brown, Boston.

Maxwell, E.K. (1986) 'Fading out: resource control and cross-cultural patterns of deference', *Journal of Cross-Cultural Gerontology* 1(1): 73–90.

Myerhoff, B. (1984) 'Rites and signs of ripening: the intertwining of time ritual, time and growing older', in D. Kertzer and J. Keith (eds) *Age and Anthropological Theory*, London: Cornell University Press.

Rosow, I. (1967) *Social Integration of the Aged*, New York: Free Press.

Stephens, J.B. (1976) *Loners, Losers and Lovers*, Seattle: University of Washington Press.

Streib, G. (1976) 'Social stratification and ageing', in R. Binstock and E. Shanas (eds) *Handbook of Ageing and the Social Sciences*, New York: Van Nostrand.

Unruh, D. (1983) *Invisible Lives*, California: Sage.

Vesperi, M.D. (1985) *City of Green Benches*, Ithaca: Cornell University Press.

Williams, R. (1986) 'Images of age and generation', unpublished paper prepared for British Sociological Association conference, Loughborough, UK.

Chapter nine

Support Networks in Old Age: Constructing a Typology[†]

G. Clare Wenger

It is now generally accepted that most care, help, and support in old age comes from informal sources. An image of the family as an available and responsible source of support has gradually replaced an earlier stereotype of the fragmented modern family in industrial societies as unavailable and unconcerned with the plight of its older generations (Lebowitz 1980). Despite this realization, however, anxieties have persisted about that minority of old people for whom such help appeared not to be available (for example, Abrams 1978), particularly those who were childless and/or living alone. Recently, more attention has been paid to the potential role of neighbours, i.e. non-kin, in the lives of elderly people (Bulmer 1986).

As research on family relationships in old age became more sophisticated, the specifics of precisely who provided help, what kinds of help were forthcoming and how often elderly people had contacts with members of their families received considerable attention, but usually such studies focused on relationships with adult children or less frequently on brothers and sisters or grandchildren. Other relatives were hardly considered and non-kin relationships received rare attention. Research on the totality of the support networks formed by involved family, friends, and neighbours has been conducted in the UK only in the last decade (Sinclair *et al.* 1984; Wenger 1984.)

Early network studies focused on such structural aspects as the size, density, and linkages of support networks, analysing variation in terms of intervening variables (age, gender, and marital status), but less attention has been given to different types of networks based on differences in membership and composition. Such variation results in different expectations and obligations in terms of the provision of help and support. This chapter, therefore, seeks to differentiate between types of support networks and to draw attention to the significance of differences for

[†] This chapter is a shortened version of a longer paper, the full version of which can be obtained from the author on request.

service provision. In this context, the *support* network is specifically differentiated from the larger *social* network, of which it forms the core, and consists of all those who are available to an elderly person to provide companionship, help, advice, support, or personal care in a regular way. Following a brief review of the findings of earlier network research, five different types of support network are identified and described, and the predictive value of these categories is then discussed.

Review of earlier network research

Network research in the UK has been limited and most of the data on support networks, discussed here, come from the USA. Comparisons with the UK must, therefore, be cautious.

Size and density

Active social networks are made up of an average of 16–50 persons but most people receive help from a minority of those who are close to them. In emergencies, approximately one-third may be counted upon for help, but fewer will help with daily needs (Wellman 1981). In the US, retired people have the lowest numbers of helpers (Warren 1981). Despite this, research has shown that most old people have a core of others available to them which, in Western society, seems to follow a similar size and distribution. Studies from the US (Stephens *et al.* 1978), Australia (Mugford and Kendig 1986), and the UK (Wenger 1984) have all found that on average elderly people have 5–7 members in their support networks.

Closely related to size is the question of density. Density refers to the proportion of members of a network known to one another. Density has actually been measured infrequently in the study of total social networks. Support networks made up of those involved with one particular elderly person will typically be of high density, since the majority of members will live in close proximity to the person in whose support they are involved. High-density support networks have been shown to be well-integrated, solidary groupings (Wellman 1981). They are generally small with strong linkages and are likely to provide strong emotional support (Craven and Wellman 1973). Low density networks are more likely to be larger, more fragmented, and heterogeneous (Wellman 1981), but may provide better access to tangible resources (Craven and Wellman 1973) by maximizing communication channels. Members of loose-knit or low-density networks may, therefore, be better able to secure help, although such help may be less reliable (Wellman 1981). Small dense networks appear to hinder the flow of knowledge (d'Abbs 1982), and there is some evidence to suggest that members of close-knit, dense networks are less likely to seek help from formal services (McKinlay 1973). Urbanism tends to reduce density, as does middle-class status (Fischer 1977a).

Diversified networks have greater potential in help-seeking and making new contacts (d'Abbs 1982); so density is not associated with the availability of social support. Most *social* networks in the west are loosely-knit, but despite this most people have intimate ties with both family and friends (Wellman 1979). Different kinds of networks are also related to different types of help-seeking behaviour (Warren 1981; Craven and Wellman 1973).

Linkages

Size and density refer to the *numbers* of members and the numbers of the links between them. Links between members may be uniplex, involving only one form of content, for instance, cousin; or multiplex, involving more than one form of content, for example, cousin, friend, and source of transport. Multiple linkages are stronger and are more likely to be reciprocal. The support networks of the elderly tend to have a core of highly multiplex relations (for example, daughter, cook, source of emotional support, and member of household) and a periphery of less multiplex relations (for example, a neighbour who comes once a week to give a lift to church) (Mugford and Kendig 1986). Ties are affected by physical and mental health (d'Abbs 1982). Those who are mentally ill tend to develop fewer multiplex ties, i.e. less reciprocal and more superficial ties, than those who are not (Tolsdorf 1976).

In western culture ties tend to be assymetrical, with one partner benefiting more than another at any one time. All ties, however, are *potential* sources of support. They also vary in intensity. Generally speaking the stronger the tie, the more likely it is to become a source of support; and the closer the relationship the more likely it is that help will be *sought* (Wellman 1979, 1981).

Content and composition

Most members of the support and social networks of elderly people are family and a high proportion is middle-aged or older (Mugford and Kendig 1986, Wenger 1986). The kin network provides a source of both mutual aid and sociability. Aid is not restricted to emergencies, but mutual aid is most common within the parent/child/sibling core. It is from this axis that aid is more frequently sought, offered, and provided, although in emergencies other parts of the family and non-kin may become involved. Family aid is sought most frequently in the context of sickness. With increasing age and/or dependency, more reliance on the family develops (Wenger 1986).

Intervening variables

Several aspects of networks are affected by gender, marital status, social class, and state of health. Women, on the whole, have larger networks than men, with more bonds with friends and siblings and more multiplex ties (Mugford and Kendig 1986). Women are also more likely to have intimate same-sex friends (Wellman 1981; Corin 1982). While the networks of both men and women are family based, women's networks are more likely to have extra-familial bonds (Corin 1982).

Elderly men's networks tend to be more polarized — that is, more focused on their children (where they have them) — and more tied to their own neighbourhood, as well as being smaller than women's.

Living with a spouse only is linked to smaller networks for elderly women but larger networks for men (ibid). Spouses play a central part in helping networks (Warren 1981). Married people, on the whole, have larger networks than those who are unmarried or widowed, although widowed women maintain larger networks (Mugford and Kendig 1986). Results from the author's first survey suggested that men's networks shrink on widowhood while women's remain stable (Wenger 1984).

The networks of the single have been shown to be more self-sufficient (ibid.; Mugford and Kendig 1986). Single women typically have large networks of siblings, friends, and neighbours, but they find it more difficult to remain in the community with advancing age (Mugford and Kendig 1986) because they are less likely to have a close relative able to provide a high level of support.

Social class also has an effect on networks as a result of differential resources and geographical mobility. Amongst the middle class there is extensive mutual aid and financial help (d'Abbs 1982). Middle-class networks are more affected by migration, therefore more widely dispersed, but also less constrained by distance (ibid.). They have greater access to transport and telephones. Middle-class networks are also more heterogeneous. The middle class establish relationships more quickly, are less likely to turn to family, and more inclined to turn to friends for help (Warren 1981).

The working-class elderly, on the other hand, have small social networks; these are kin dominated (Mugford and Kendig 1986), the mother-daughter link being especially strong (d'Abbs 1982). Working-class networks tend to have more intense ties with neighbours (Warren 1981). Working-class people appear to be more seriously affected before seeking help, especially extra-familial help (Warren 1981).

The availability of supportive ties does not appear to be related to health (Wellman 1981), but those who are more dependent are likely to have a higher proportion of family members in their networks, and

169

for them ties with less closely related kin seem to be more important (Mugford and Kendig 1986).

Orientations to networks and help-seeking

People have different perspectives towards their networks. While most people resolve their problems by drawing on informal sources, some feel more comfortable about asking for help than others. Those who have positive attitudes towards their support networks feel that it is safe, advisable and necessary to confide in other people and to ask for help or advice when needed. Others, whose attitudes towards their networks have been described as negative, regard their networks with some distrust or suspicion, feeling that asking for help or confiding is inadvisable, impossible or pointless. Those who suffer from some form of mental illness are particularly likely to adopt the latter orientation (Tolsdorf 1976).

Personality and social skills affect the structure and function of networks (Mugford and Kendig 1986). It has been noted that those with a positive orientation ask for and receive more network support. Attitudes towards the network also affect its development, with those whose attitudes are positive and trusting developing more multiplex linkages and reciprocal ties. Where attitudes are negative or suspicious of others, for instance in cases of depression or paranoia, potential helpers may withdraw or curtail involvement (Tolsdorf 1976).

Help-seeking is mediated through the network, which affects access to resources, whereas the ability to cope with crises is related to the structure and nature of the network (d'Abbs 1982). Coping strategies are also likely to be related to physical health or other problems. Those who have more control over their situation are likely to develop a diversified coping style, while those who suffer frequent or severe crises tend to adopt a concentrated style, relying on one or two close members of the family or friends (d'Abbs 1982).

Help-seeking, it has been suggested, goes against western societal values of independence and self-reliance, although fewer constraints exist for the very young and the very old (Warren 1981; Weeks and Cuellar 1981).

Different types of networks

The preceding paragraphs have highlighted some of the factors which contribute to variation in social as well as support networks. So far, attempts to devise network typologies have been limited, primarily due to the complexity of the methodology necessary to look at networks as entities. Typologies based on survey data, therefore, tend to be based on one or a few simple criteria.

170

Methodology

The data presented in this chapter come from the first and second phases of a longitudinal study funded by the Department of Health and Social Security (DHSS) and since 1986 by the ESRC. The study consisted primarily of three surveys conducted in 1979, 1983, and 1987, during which elderly people were interviewed in their own homes. (N (1979) = 534). As part of phase II of the research, thirty people, who had been over 75 years old when the study started in 1979, were studied intensively from 1983 to 1986, by which time they were already in their eightieth year or older. It is from this intensive small sample study that the data on which this chapter is based originate.

The intensive phase of the study made possible the collection of a wide range of data on support networks. While interest was centred on the *support* network, data were gradually collected on the active *social* network by recording the details of all other members of the wider network mentioned by each old person in the course of lengthy discussions. Over the months from 1983 to 1986 a picture was built up of the other important relationships in the lives of the elderly people participating in this study, so that the support networks came to be perceived within a wider context. It must be stressed that any typology based on a sample of thirty old people must remain tentative. However, my own anthropological perspective leads me to believe that careful, detailed analysis of small samples are at least as valid (and probably more so) as is bare statistical analysis of numerical variables in large-scale studies. The face validity of small-scale network studies, originated by Bott (1957), is by now well recognized, as is the importance of participant-observation in network analysis (Wellman 1979).

Network typology

On the basis of detailed data from the intensive study, five fairly distinctive types of support network were identified, which on the basis of the old persons' relationships to their networks, I have called:

(1) *The local integrated support network*, typically including close relationships with local family, friends, and neighbours; usually based on long-established residence and active community involvement in the present or recent past.

(2) *The local self-contained support network*, typically have arms-length relationships or infrequent contact, if any, with local kin, relying mainly on neighbours. Respondents are characterized by a retiring nature and largely privatized household-centred lifestyle. Community involvement, if there is any, is low key.

(3) *The wider-community-focused support network*, typically including distant kin, with high salience of friends, some neighbours; characterized by high level of community activities and involvement, usually associated with absence of local kin.

(4) *The family-dependent support network*, having primary focus on close local family ties with few peripheral friends or neighbours. These are often based on shared household with, or living close to, adult child (usually a daughter).

(5) *The private restricted support network*, characterized by absence of local kin, other than spouse in some cases, and limited contact with local community. No local friends and superficial contact with neighbours.

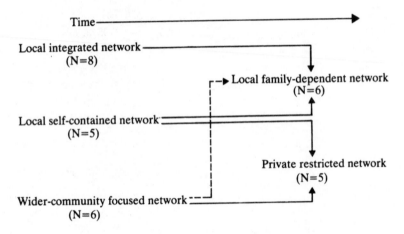

The arrows signify possible developments rather than inevitable change. The dotted arrow indicates a possible development which only occurs where a move is involved.

Figure 9.1 Support network typology — Increased dependency with passage of time

There was evidence in the intensive study to demonstrate that the family-dependent (type 4) and the private-restricted network (type 5) may (but do not necessarily) develop out of other types, as indicated in Figure 9.1. In a larger sample, it is possible that other shifts might also be identified. Shifts of this type (which are discussed subsequently) do not necessarily reflect change in the size or composition of the network so much as the effects of the ageing process on respondents and network members.

Other network studies of different types of households suggest some common or comparable features with those which underlie this typology. Bott's study (1957) was focused on couples and her primary interest was conjugal roles, but there are in her study obvious parallels with the support networks of the elderly. More recently, other authors have written about the relationships between network type and helping behaviours, also based on couples or families with children (Price 1984; Brannen 1985).

Figure 9.2 illustrates in diagram form the relationships between the various typologies. The fact that parallels exist reinforces the validity of the distinctions. The comparability between networks at earlier stages of the life cycle and those after 75 suggests that broadly the typology holds with age.

Bott (1957) N=20	*Price* (1984) N=40	*Brannen* (1985) N=48	*Wenger* (1987a, b) N=30
Close-knit	Local solidaristic (a) Kin-centred (b) Neighbour-centered	Close-knit	Local integrated Family-dependent
Medium-knit			
	Household Family	Truncated	Local self-contained
Transitional			
			Private restricted
Loose-knit	Familiar Associate	Extended/ segmented	Community-focused

Figure 9.2 Comparison of network typologies

Each of the typologies: (1) reflects a continuum from close-knit or high density, to loose-knit or low density; (2) identifies the correlations with social class; and (3) acknowledges the influence of neighbour-hood. Bott's scheme focuses on the degree of connectedness or density, rather than on help-seeking and help-receiving behaviours. While all the schemes have comparable network types at the extremes of the continua, there is less similarity with Bott between these poles.

In short, the typology of support networks of elderly people is broadly consistent with earlier network classification. The parallels suggest that it is possible to identify types of help-seeking behaviour based on network type. Certainly, the indications are that an understanding of network type would make it easier to predict and understand patterns of demand for help.

The defining characteristics of the elderly support networks are: the availability and proximity of family members, the categories of family members available locally, and the degree of involvement demonstrated by the respondents with family, friends, neighbours, and community. In addition to observable differences in network structure and composition, the categories also demonstrate overall differences in terms of their average radius, density, numbers of support ties, the proportion of ties with members of the family, and the size of the larger *social* as opposed to *support* network, summarized in Table 9.1 and discussed at greater length in subsequent paragraphs.

Support networks followed a bi-modal distribution in terms of their radii, with networks tending to be locally based, i.e. located within five miles, or dispersed, i.e. with at least one member more than twenty-five miles away. Usually, those members of support networks who lived at a distance were adult children whose support was sought in crises despite distance and who were still likely to be the relative seen most often. It might be anticipated in the context of the support network in small communities that density would be high. However, while the average density was 0.75, measured density in this study of the support networks of elderly people ranged from 1.00, in which all members knew one another, down to 0.33.

Support networks also differed in terms of the number of support ties which existed in the network, as measured by the numbers of times a respondent listed a member of the network in any support role — for instance, members of the household, helpers in various situations, and so on. The number of ties listed was affected by personality, level of disability or social isolation. Larger numbers of ties indicated either high levels of dependency or of gregariousness. The proportion of ties to family members also varied in terms of available family, both by size of family and proximity of family members. On the whole, however, the figure reflects the involvement or lack of involvement with friends and neighbours in the community.

Data analysed and presented elsewhere (Wenger 1987a) demonstrate that a hierarchy of relationships exists, which not only reflects the relative importance of different categories of relationship, but which also follows a continuum in terms of frequency of contact, salience in the old person's life, and the level of commitment and involvement likely to occur on the basis of normative expectations and responsibilities. At the top of the hierarchy are spouses, followed by adult children. Also, different types of networks tend to have different types of relationship in their membership.

Table 9.1 Summary of network typology. Mean statistics

Type of network	Age	Size of support network	Radius (miles)	No. in one mile	Density	No. of Ties	% family ties	No. of kin	No. of Friends	No. of Neighbours	No. in Social Network
Local integrated N=8	82.6 (80–87)	8.4 (6–11)	<15	5.9	0.81	22.0	65	4.5	1.6	1.5	20
Local self-contained N=5	81.0 (79–83)	6.0 (3–10)	<9	3.6	0.83	14.0	45	3.0	0.6	2.0	16
Family dependent N=6	84.2 (81–92)	5.6 (3–8)	<13	4.3	0.74	23.5	87	4.0	1.2	0.8	16
Private-restricted N=5	87.5 (83–95)	5.8 (2–10)	>25	3.0	0.68	17.5	47	3.0	1.0	1.4	15
Wider Community-focused N=6	81.7 (79–85)	7.5 (4–11)	>25	4.5	0.69	24.4	50	3.5	2.5	1.2	27
Overall N=30	83.3	7.0		3.96	0.75	20.6	60	3.6	1.4	14	18

The five identified network categories are, of course, ideal types. There were a few individuals whose networks did not fit easily into any one category, but it is possible to characterize the different types of networks as follows.

1. The local integrated support network

Local integrated networks typically included involved local family, often both immediate and extended, and local friends and/or neighbours. The eight old people with this type of network were either still involved in a range of community activities, or had been in the recent past. They were usually long-term residents who had either raised their families in their present community or had lived there during their childhood. They were likely to have relatives of both their own generation and younger generations living locally and to be well-known to other members of the community, so that most, if not all, linkages were multiplex. Support network membership in this category was marginally larger than those in others (average size 8+) and of high density (average 0.81), indicative of a high level of integration.

On average, respondents in this category had the largest numbers of members in the support network living within a mile and the highest number of family members of the support network. Friends and neighbours were important. Their day-to-day lives involved frequent contacts with others. Their networks were likely to reflect a large number of support ties, i.e. linkage to someone providing some aspect of support, (average 22, range 17–29) and an overall high reliance on family (65% of ties). Most ties were with support network members living within five miles.

Their *social* networks tended to be large and active, mainly made up of extended family but including local friends and neighbours. They typically relied mainly on a member of a younger generation living in a separate household. Six of the eight were judged to have markedly warm, outgoing personalities and all but one a well-developed sense of humour. The use of formal services tended to be delayed until disability was acute.

2. The local self-contained support network

This network differed from the previous one primarily in terms of the patterns of involvement in it of the old people themselves. The five people with this network type seemed to share some similarity of personality: typically shy or retiring by nature, satisfied with their own company, and adopting privatized life-styles with little expectation of help from others. They were all childless, although three had married. None of them had played active roles in local community groups at any stage of their life, although all belonged to a church or chapel. Participation, when it occurred, however, tended to be low key. All had relatives or their spouse's relatives, mainly siblings, cousins, nieces, or nephews, living nearby, but in only one case could the family relationship be characterized as involved.

These support networks were typically smaller (average size 6) than the local integrated type, although equally dense (0.83). They were also likely to have all members within a five-mile radius, although the average number of members within a mile was low (3.6) and they were likely to have a low number of support ties (average 14, range 3–21), reflecting their basic independence from others. There was also more reliance on neighbours with an average of only 45% of ties with family.

Their social networks were typically comparatively small and limited to local extended kin, and they tended to have a household orientation.

Those in this category represent a vulnerable group, and the fact that their average age, at 81, was the lowest of all categories reflects the fact that members of this group, because they are least likely to be able to rally assistance, are more likely to enter residential care.

3. The wider-community-focused support network

In contrast to the two preceding network types, most of the six persons in this network type were unlikely to have local family. They were also more likely to have moved to the community from elsewhere on retirement or during middle age. None had children living locally and all had support networks with radii of more than twenty-five miles, including children who were psychologically important members. All those with this type of network were in relatively good health, most were middle class and all were involved with friends and neighbours and active in local organizations. All had outgoing, friendly personalities and self-confidence. This type of network was concentrated in communities with high retirement migration.

Networks of this type were slightly larger than average (average 7.5) and, not unexpectedly, of lower density (average 0.69). The average age was 82. The average number of support ties was high (average 24.4, range 15–28), indicative more of involvement than dependency; and despite distance, 50 per cent of ties were with family. Ties by telephone and rapid transport were important. Independence was jealously protected, but help was accepted when *they* decided it was necessary. Involvement with local friends and neighbours was high, and social networks were extensive. Visits to and from distant family and friends were common, and distant links were maintained as a matter of course.

4. The local family-dependent support network

This network describes a situation in which the old person relies on close family for most needs. Of the six people with this type of network, five lived with a female relative and one in a granny-flat at her son's home. They maintained few local contacts beyond the household, although all had one or two support ties outside the household. As a result these networks were smaller (average 5.6, range 3–8). Surprisingly, the density of these networks is not as high as one might anticipate (0.74), primarily because non-local kin to whom old people might turn for advice, for instance, tended not to know local contacts outside the household.

Most of those in this category were very dependent as a result of which the number of support ties is high (average 23.5, range 19–29). The larger social network tended to be limited to the extended family with some superficial contact with neighbours or children's friends.

It is difficult to comment fairly on personality since all of these old people were already very dependent when I met them; but all appeared to expect to be taken care of, some indicating that their expectations were not being met as well as they would wish! Involvement of community nursing was highest in this category.

5. The private restricted support network

This network was characterized by an absence of local family, other than in some cases a spouse, and limited contact with the local community. None had close local friends and contacts with neighbours were perfunctory. In some instances, the old person had outlived local friends. Three out of the five old people with this type of network were childless. Only two could rely on family support, even from a distance. Reflecting this, networks were slightly smaller than average (averaging 5.8, range 2–10), less dense (0.68), and all had radii over twenty-five miles.

Despite a high average age (87.5), these old people had low numbers of support ties (average 17.5), reflecting not only the paucity of support but also the determined independence that they all demonstrated. Despite the lack of available family support, an average of 47 per cent of support ties were with family; however, this group demonstrated a heavy reliance on domiciliary services, particularly home help and meals-on-wheels. Social networks tended to be limited to long-distance perfunctory contacts with extended family. The vulnerability of the elderly with networks of this type is self-evident.

Based on the evidence of this small sample, the identified support-network types appeared to be fairly evenly distributed in the elderly population, with one-third having networks which left them vulnerable. The effects of gender on network formation are reflected in the typology in the finding that men were overrepresented in the two most vulnerable categories, the local self-contained and the private restricted networks. Half those in these two categories were men, whereas they constituted only one-third of the total sample. The importance of marital status was also reflected in the findings: four of the five who had never married had networks in the two most vulnerable categories. Family structure was also important. Those in the family dependent category were slightly more likely than those with networks in other categories to have daughters, while two-thirds of the childless had support networks identified as vulnerable — that is, either local self-contained or private restricted.

Conclusions: the predictive significance of types of support network

The findings indicate that different types of support network exist among elderly people living in the community, depending on: the availability of local family; the specific family relationships available (i.e. daughters and sisters or nieces and cousins); the closeness of ties with local family; and the patterns of interaction which old people develop with the larger community of friends, neighbours, and voluntary groups, mediated through the personality of the respondent.

Changes in the caring capacity of the network appear to be related to the death, increasing frailty, or other changes in the circumstances of members, or to shifts in network type due to the inexorable passage of time, rather than in the refusal, reluctance, or alienation of network members. Networks with few younger generation members are more vulnerable than those which contain them.

Different types of support network reflect different combinations of relationships, and different relationships include different normative expectations and responsibilities, so that one might expect that different kinds of network meet different kinds of need more effectively than others. At the same time, different types of neighbourhood are likely to reflect different distributions of network types. If this is so and we know the distribution of support network types within a neighbourhood, we should be better able to predict what needs are likely to be unmet and, therefore, what problems are likely to be present.

Those with *local integrated support networks* tend to have larger networks than most other old people and have more contact with a wider range of relationships. They are likely to maintain relationships with both immediate and extended family and to be more involved with local friends, and with neighbours.

Social and practical support for those with this kind of network is likely to be spread throughout the network, with day-to-day contact and security provided by relationships with involved neighbours, companionship needs met by siblings or friends, and practical help and moral support also available from local relatives. High morale, positive self-image, and self-esteem are common. Professional interventions are likely to be sought only as a last resort.

For all these reasons, however, it is likely that professionals may find it both more acceptable and effective to work in partnership with this type of network. Neighbourhoods where this network type predominates are likely to accommodate paid good-neighbour schemes, quasi-formal monitoring arrangements, and other community-based collaborations with statutory services better than are less cohesive neighbourhoods. However, it may also be appropriate to encourage earlier formal intervention in such contexts, as referrals, when they come, are more likely to represent crises or intractable situations where the informal network has tried everything within its power before help is sought. Earlier intervention might pre-empt the development of crises.

In contrast, those with *local self-contained support networks* tend to keep themselves to themselves and to focus their lives on the household. They are likely to be childless and immediate family in the support network are likely to be brothers and sisters, often living at more than walking distance away. Membership of extended family in the support network is likely to be meagre, confined to nieces or nephews seen infrequently. Neighbours are more important to this group than to others and friends least in evidence. This type of network can often be described as neighbour-dependent. Social networks are primarily composed of extended family, rarely seen, with whom contacts are mainly symbolic.

If married, old people in such networks may cope well until widowed, and then they may be more severely affected by the loss of companionship than those in locally integrated or wider-community-focused types of network. The same is true for households consisting of ageing siblings, when one dies. Social isolation is more of a risk in this context, frequently exacerbated by independence in the face of growing frailty. While in good health, those with local self-contained support networks may cope well, seemingly content with lower levels of social interaction and managing with occasional help and monitoring from neighbours. Regular help is not always available, although neighbours may be helpful. However, old people in this type of network are most likely to resist help or professional intervention and, if living alone, are more likely to suffer from emergencies which are not immediately recognized as such. Professionals seeking to work with or through neighbours need to adopt a kid-glove approach; yet paradoxically, neighbours are often the first to contact agencies.

Wider-community-focused support networks are primarily friend-centred, although distant children are likely to feature as frequently in the membership. Extended family membership of the support network is likely to be low and neighbour membership confined to one or two near neighbours. Social networks are likely to be extensive rather than dense. This support network is primarily a middle-class adaptation.

High morale is common in this group. The extra-familial friendship focus is associated with a high level of companionship, and a positive self-image and self-esteem. Frequent contact with children is maintained by telephone. Help in emergencies is forthcoming both from friends and from children living at a distance. However, long-term help or support is often difficult. While many are in a position to pay for regular help, it is from this group that early requests are made to statutory agencies, often as a reflection of anxieties of distant children. Since many retirement migrants have this type of network, local care-providers often perceive retirement migration as a drain on local services.. Evidence, not used here, however, demonstrates that a higher proportion of long-term than of immigrant residents receives services (Wenger 1984).

Early requests for help, moreover, could result in early interventions which could obviate later crises. Help with problem-solving by adopting a broker role is likely to be appropriate in neighbourhoods where community-focused networks predominate: for example, assistance in recruiting private help is a coping device which would be welcomed by some old people.

Those with *family-dependent support networks* are likely to be older and more frail than others and to rely primarily on members of the immediate family. In most cases, this means a daughter. In all such cases in the study, the old person was living in a shared household with a daughter, son or sister. These networks can also occur where members of the immediate family live nearby. Contacts with friends and neighbours are usually peripheral, reflecting merely contacts via the caring relative. That individual tends to be the focus of all the help needed or demanded. Larger social networks consist primarily of extended family.

Old people in this network type, cared for by daughters in shared households, can expect support in excess of the normative expectations for adult children. They receive regular help with the activities of daily life and with personal care if needed. In terms of practical help and support such old people receive a high quality of care.

Because contacts beyond the immediate household are peripheral, however, regular social contact with other family members tends to be restricted and with younger generations when it occurs. It is not surprising, therefore, to find that loneliness is common amongst those living with their children (Wenger 1984), whose contact with age peers is limited.

Where the old person is living with a sibling the need for companionship and mutual support can lead to a mutually satisfying relationship until one becomes dependent on the other.

Those family-dependent support networks centred on non-married daughters are likely to be the most durable, because they do not involve conflicting responsibilities for a spouse (in this age-group often retired). Siblings are less likely to continue to care in the face of high dependency. However, where the dependent sibling has been a surrogate parent earlier in the life cycle, the expectations for children appear to be met (Wenger 1987a).

Those with this network type, therefore, may expect continuing practical help and moral support with increasing frailty. However, while physical needs are met, friendship needs may not be. In contrast, those living with or cared for by siblings (usually a sister) are likely to have higher morale; but continued practical care may be fragile due not only to the greater age of carers, but to the mismatch of normative expectations.

In this context, it is important to note that shared households established specifically to accommodate the increasing frailty of a parent are an exception to the rule, and they are more likely to experience strain than those established before the onset of dependency. Most of the latter were originally based on reciprocity, and have established an expectation of care provision when the parent ages (Wenger 1987b).

The implications for health and social services in the context of this type of network suggest the importance of recognition of the focus of demand on one (usually female) member of the immediate family, thus concentrating responsibility and, in cases of high dependence, strain. In most cases, such networks manage well until the strain of demands, often exacerbated by mental illness of the old person or by the physical illness of the carer, results in a request for help. Recognizing the normative expectations for the relationship can indicate appropriate intervention (Wenger 1987a). Thus, for example, assessments and interventions relating to the mental health of either the old person or the carer may be more appropriate in cases where the carers are children, and practical help where the carers are siblings.

Above all, it is important to recognize that expectations are culturally defined: reluctance or inability to exceed expectations is not usually indicative of lack of concern or inadequacy on the part of members of the family. Professional care providers need to understand normative expectations in order to appreciate what it is reasonable to expect from a specific relative in a specific situation (ibid). Daughters tend to ask for help only as a last resort, while siblings need and may ask for help sooner.

The *private restricted support network* is characterized by the absence of local kin and infrequent, arms-length contacts with local people who may be defined by the old person as friends or neighbours. These networks, together with the family-dependent support networks, contain the fewest members. Old people with this type of network, unless their spouses are still alive, suffer lack of companionship and an absence of informal practical help. Emergency help is rarely forthcoming from family, and neighbour monitoring is likely to be the only local input. Half of those with networks of this type relied primarily on statutory services, but while practical help and personal care came from these sources, help with loneliness and resulting depression was absent.

To summarize, depending on the type of their support network, old people in the community have access to different sorts of support. Those with family-dependent support networks may be expected to receive a high level of practical help and support, but may be isolated from important contact with age peers or extra-familial contacts. Those with local integrated support networks are likely to be well supported, both practically and emotionally, and thus to have high morale, especially if they are still married or have children in the same community. Similarly, those with wider community-focused support networks are likely to have good emotional support and high morale. However, long-term, practical support is likely to be problematic. Those with local self-contained or private restricted support networks are likely to be most at risk. Neither have frequent contacts with family, although the former are likely to have some friendly contacts with neighbours. Neither include relationships involving expectations of emotional support or regular practical help (ibid).

Areas with high proportions of middle-class, geographically mobile households will have higher proportions of wider community-focused support networks. They are likely to occur in areas of high retirement migration. Stable market towns, on the other hand, are likely to have a larger proportion of locally integrated support networks. The distribution of network types between communities has obvious implications for community styles of intervention. The distribution of different relationships within an individual's support network provides important indications of the kinds of support which can be expected in the future. Understanding the variation in support networks and the incidence of network types in the community, therefore, provide important pointers for the caring professional and local policy-maker in planning interventions at both case and community levels.

References

d'Abbs, P. (1982) *Social Support Networks: A Critical review of Models and Findings*, Melbourne: Institute of Family Studies Monograph No. 1.

Abrams, M. (1978) *Beyond Three-score and Ten: A First Report on a Survey of the Elderly*, London: Age Concern.

Bott, E. (1957) *Family and Social Network*, London: Tavistock Institute of Human Relations.

Brannen, J. (1985) 'Suitable cases for treatment? Couples seeking help for marital difficulties', in J. Brannen and G. Wilson (eds) *Support Networks in a Caring Community*, Lancaster: Kluwer Academic Publishers, pp. 125–38.

Bulmer, M. (1986) *Neighbours: The Work of Philip Abrams*, Cambridge: Cambridge University Press.

Corin, E. (1982) 'Elderly people's social strategies for survival: a dynamic use of social networks analysis', *Canada's Mental Health* 30(3): 7–12.

Craven, P. and Wellman, B. (1973) 'The network city', *Sociological Inquiry* 43 (3–4): 57–88.

Fischer, C.S. (1977a) 'Network analysis and urban studies', in Claude S. Fischer *et al.*, *Networks and Places: Social Relations in the Urban Setting*, New York: Free Press, pp. 19–37.

Fischer, C.S. (1977b) 'Perspectives on community and personal relations', in Claude S. Fischer *et al.*, *Networks and Places: Social Relations in the Urban Setting*, New York: Free Press, pp. 1–16.

Lebowitz, B.D. (1980) 'Old age and family functioning', *Journal of Geronotological Social Work* 1(2): 111–18.

McKinlay, J. (1973) 'Social networks, lay consultation and help-seeking behaviour', *Social Forces* 51: 275–92.

Mugford, S. and Kendig, H. (1986) 'Social relations: networks and ties', in H. Kendig (ed.) *Ageing and Families: A Social Networks Perspective*, Sydney: Allen and Unwin, pp. 38–59.

Price, F. (1984) 'Making Connections: Mothers as Mediators for "Family" and "School" ', unpublished PhD dissertation, University of Lancaster.

Sinclair, I., Crosbie, D., O'Connor, P., Stanforth, L., and Vickery, A. (1984) *Networks Project: A Study of Informal Care, Services and Social Work for Elderly Clients Living Alone*, London: National Institute for Social Work.

Stephens, R.C., Blau, Z., Oser, G., and Millar, M. (1978) 'Aging, social support systems and social policy', *Journal of Gerontological Social Work* 1(4): 33–45.

Tolsdorf, C.C. (1976) 'Social networks, support and coping: an exploratory study', *Family Process* 15: 407–17.

Warren, D.I. (1981) *Helping Networks: How People Cope with Problems in the Urban Community*, Indiana: University of Notre Dame.

Weeks, J. and Cuellar, J. (1981) 'The role of family members in the helping networks of older people', *The Gerontologist* 21: 388–94.

Wellman, B. (1979) 'The community question: the intimate networks of East Yorkers', *American Journal of Sociology* 84(5): 1201–31.

Wellman, B. (1981) 'Applying network analysis to the study of support', in B.H. Gottlieb (ed.) *Social Networks and Social Support*, Beverly Hills: Sage Publications, pp. 171–200.

Wenger, G.C. (1984) *The Supportive Network: Coping with Old Age*, London: George Allen and Unwin.

Wenger, G.C. (1986) 'A longitudinal study of changes and adaptations in the support networks of Welsh elderly over 75', *Journal of Cross-cultural Gerontology* 1(3): 277–304.

Wenger, G.C. (1987a) *Relationships in Old Age — Inside Support Networks: Third Report of a Follow-up Study of Old Elderly People in North Wales*, Bangor, Gwynedd: Report to DHSS/Welsh Office, Centre for Social Policy Research and Development, University College of North Wales.

Wenger, G.C. (1987b) 'Dependence, independence and reciprocity after 80', *Journal of Ageing Studies* 1(4): 355–77.

Chapter ten

Contested Territory in Informal Care[†]

Jane Lewis and Barbara Meredith

Introduction

The importance of the role of informal carers of the elderly has been widely acknowledged in the 1980s. In its 1981 White Paper, *Growing Older*, government expressed both its faith in the existence of a pool of carers ready and willing to assume family care responsibilities and its view that formal (state-financed) and informal care constitute alternative systems, rather than points on a single spectrum of provision for elderly people (Parliamentary Paper 1981). In the 1981 document informal care was promoted over formal care both for reasons of cost-saving and because it was felt that the effort to underpin informal care by state-financed provision ran the risk of introducing rigidities into the informal system, thereby destroying its chief virtue: 'It is the role of public authorities to sustain and, where necessary develop — but never to displace — such support and care. Care *in* the community must increasingly mean care *by* the community' (ibid.: 3).

Academic research has subjected the idea of the formal and informal sectors as alternatives to considerable scrutiny. Above all, clear evidence of the crucial role played by professional supporters in relieving informal carer strain has been adduced (see especially Levin *et al.* 1983). Increasingly, attention has focused on the ways in which caring might be 'shared', how a 'partnership' might be developed, or how 'interweaving' might be achieved (Bayley 1973; Hadley 1981; Bulmer 1986). Many demonstration projects have focused particularly on the possible role for a 'third force' in the forms of 'volunteerism and neighbourhoodism' (Davies and Challis 1986) and the ways in which such a pool of carers may be linked to the formal and informal systems. As the Audit Commission (1986) report on community care has commented, policy in the field has been characterized largely by muddling

---

[†] This chapter is a shortened version of a longer paper, the full version of which can be obtained from the authors on request.

through. However, the recent literature and growing number of pilot projects, many of which as yet have received no formal evaluation (see Cloke 1985; Chambers 1986) suggest a vigorous commitment to exploring different ways of constructing care packages drawing on informal, voluntary, and formal supporters, and combining different methods of financing (Leat and Gay 1987).

The dimensions of the problem are such that diverse experimentation is warranted. The Equal Opportunities Commission has estimated that there are already one-and-a quarter million informal carers (the vast majority of them women) (EOC 1982). By the year 2001 the number of over 75s — the age-group commonly agreed to be in need of most care — is projected to rise by 30 per cent and the number of over 85s almost to double (Ermisch 1983; Wicks and Henwood 1984). However, while there is no question but that we need to be more imaginative in constructing ways of supporting elderly people and their informal supporters, the language of 'sharing', 'partnership', and 'interweaving' tend to minimize the possibility of conflict and contested territory. This is all the more surprising in view of the boundary that has existed historically between the public and private spheres and which recent New Right writing on the family has sought to reinforce (for example, Mount 1983). Our small-scale qualitative study of the caring process suggests that more attention needs to be given to the difficulties that might arise from attempting to construct different kinds of care packages for elderly people living at home. Although our research revealed instances of caring and knowledgable support for carers at home, these were rare and it is our hope that our findings will contribute especially to the development of a carer-centred approach, which is being developed by some innovative schemes such as the Kent Community Care scheme (Davies and Challis 1986).

The study

In the Spring of 1986 we undertook an exploratory project, interviewing forty-one women who had cared for their mothers on a co-resident basis, in order to examine the natural history of the caring process. The number of elderly living with kin has fallen dramatically from about 42 per cent in the early 1960s to 20 per cent at the beginning of the 1980s, although, as Willmott (1986) points out, between two-thirds and three-quarters of all elderly people living at home still see relatives at least once a week. Relationships between elderly people and kin still require frequent, often difficult, often painful, negotiation.

Of the forty-one daughter respondents, twenty-nine were single, nine married, one widowed, and one divorced. In all but three cases caring had ceased within the last ten years, because the mother had either entered an institution or died. General Household Survey (GHS) data for 1980 showed that of all carers, 8 per cent were single daughters and 11 per cent married daughters. Our sample therefore appears skewed towards the single-daughter carer. This is explained in part by the derivation of the sample[1] — many of the respondents were obtained through contact with the National Council for Carers and their Elderly Dependants, which used to be an organization for single-women carers — and in part because most of the respondents belonged to a cohort that reached maturity during or just after the Second World War, when the proportion of never-married women was much greater than it is at the present time, and when it was much more commonly expected that a single daughter would care for parents. While in the future there are likely to be fewer never-married carers such as these, the GHS data show that at present single women continue to provide a disproportionate number of carers relative to their numbers in the population (Evandrou *et al.* 1986).

Almost three-quarters of the respondents were in their fifties and sixties. The social class of respondents was hard to assess. Twenty-eight certainly came from middle-class backgrounds and either had professional jobs, had married middle-class men, or had continued to live in their parents' middle-class homes. Similarly, six were certainly working-class. The remainder had for the most part experienced considerable social mobility through work or marriage, but in the case of single daughters were often still living at home and identified with their working-class backgrounds.[2]

From semi-structured interviews lasting from one to three hours, we constructed 'caring biographies' through which we explored changes in the relationship between the daughters, their mothers, and significant others. We were able to identify a matrix of caring relationships. The dominant, primary caring relationship was that between mother and daughter, who also maintained to various degrees other relationships with kin, neighbours, friends, employers (in the case of daughters), and paid[3] and voluntary helpers. We were able to identify the way in which the balance between these relationships had shifted over time. As the elderly person grew increasingly physically and/or mentally dependent, her relationships with friends and even kin tended to diminish. Because caring absorbed more of the daughter's time, her extra-caring relationships also diminished: for example, she was likely to give up work. As isolation intensified, the help of paid supporters became crucial.

It is a relatively new and difficult task for paid helpers to work out ways of supporting informal carers on their home territory. Indeed, there are historical grounds for government's fear that 'expert intervention tends to result in 'take over', albeit usually only of a very specific portion of the total caring task. However, in view of carers' desire for help (articulated through studies like ours and through the voluntary organizations serving carers), the answer would seem to lie in the development of new methods of working rather than in cutting off the efforts of paid workers altogether.

In this chapter we consider the issues raised by attempts to mix formal and informal care in the setting of the home, but we also consider other less immediately obvious aspects of conflict that are part of the informal caring process and which bear upon any assessment paid workers may make of the situation. Informal care is usually considered to be preferable to institutional care because it is more flexible and more responsive to the needs of the person cared for; the principal assumption behind this belief is that care stems from altruism and love. Following Graham (1983), our definition of caring comprises more than simply 'helping', 'tending', or 'managing'. Most of our respondents experienced caring as hard physical labour and loving attention. Inevitably, ambivalent feelings arise from a role which encompasses both labour and love, and which, for many women, is both activity and identity. In turn, moreover, tension and conflict may characterize the relationship between carer and person cared for, and between carer and kin, sometimes leaving a legacy of bitterness. In the case of neighbours and friends, careful boundaries may be drawn on both sides as to what help is appropriate and as to how far they may 'penetrate' the home.

We suggest first that it cannot be assumed that 'interweaving' care merely involves the relatively simple process of identifying and filling gaps. There may well be no consensus on what the gaps are and how they might be filled: on whether it is emotional or practical support that is sought and from what source it may be found. Second, we urge a more primary-caring-relationship-centred approach. It is incumbent on the paid supporters to be aware of the variety of ways in which the home as a locus of caring can become territory contested by the carer and the person cared for, and whether the carer considers it appropriate to seek and accept help. The on-going process of negotiation between the carer and the person cared for, to which we have already referred, may extend to include implicit or explicit negotiation between one or both and potential paid supporters.

We are aware that our findings are at best generalizable to co-resident caring situations, but we believe our limited data also draw attention to the wider issue of how to achieve good working relationships between paid and informal carers in the home. The sections which follow examine first the conflicts that may develop between the carer and the person cared for, and second, the limits to the parts played by kin, neighbours, and friends in caring. Finally, we discuss the way in which paid workers come into the picture, and how the nature of other caring relationships bears upon their contribution.

Carers and persons cared for

Co-resident caring relationships are sometimes assumed to be fundament-
ally unproblematic because they are based on 'natural' feelings of love
and normative ideas of family obligations. However, as Evers (1985)
has observed, relationships between mothers and daughters are likely
to be 'fraught with ambivalence'.

From answers to questions about feelings of closeness and patterns
of communication, we assessed thirteen of the mother/daughter relationships we investigated as 'supportive' throughout the caring period,
seventeen as 'problematic' throughout, and eleven as deteriorating from
supportive to problematic. The supportive relationships, all between
unmarried daughters and their mothers, were characterized by feelings
of mutual interdependence and deep companionship. They occurred in
cases where the mother suffered physical but not mental illness; and,
although susceptible to increasing isolation as their mothers' condition
deteriorated, these daughters tended to experience less ambivalence about
caring than the remainder.

All the other relationships were characterized at some point in the
caring period by a growing imbalance, which rendered them problematic.
As the mother's physical and/or mental condition worsened, mother and
daughter often experienced tension over responsibility for routine
household tasks and later over aspects of the mother's personal care.
Matthews (1979) has described this most clearly and sympathetically in
terms of the elderly mother struggling to hold on to her sources of power
within the family. As with the daughter carers interviewed by Fisher
(1986), our respondents identified this process as one of role reversal.
In one case, for example, the mother insisted on carving the Sunday joint
long after she had relinquished responsibility for all other household tasks.
It appeared from some accounts that mothers were prepared to manipulate
the situation to assert control: one would insist on having the doctor call
and, then when he did, say there was nothing wrong with her. Such
attention-seeking behaviour was in some cases caused by painful and
isolating illness; and in others it emerged as a new phenomenon which
proved extremely wearing for carers, who, not surprisingly, reported
feeling 'trapped'. Although we relied on the daughter's perceptions of
what happened, their evidence suggests that the problems of coming to
terms with reduced capacities and the fear of dying bulk large for persons
being cared for, larger indeed than is probably realized by carers or paid
supporters.

These feelings may serve to explain a common phenomenon among
those whose relationships with their mothers became at some point
problematic, viz. the mother's apparent failure to co-operate in her care.
In these cases, the carers stated that their mothers actively resisted or

rejected specific efforts made to help them. Such an experience proved much more difficult for carers than the issue of role reversal, because not only was caring made additionally stressful, but the carer received no positive response to her efforts. In cases where the mother's behaviour was the result of dementia, the carer felt guilty if she expressed her feelings of frustration and anger.

Eighteen respondents reported some failure of their mothers to co-operate in their care. Most common was the refusal to consider the possibility of someone else caring: for instance, the mother would either refuse to have a sitter or to go into a home while the daughter went on holiday. This was often clearly the result of dementia. Faced with such a problem, the response of carers was often confused. One, for example, who had admitted her mother to a nursing home while she took a holiday, returned home after a day because her mother was distressed: 'I still felt obliged to come back, even though they got her into a nursing home, although everyone said don't.'

Some daughters managed to deal with these sorts of situations by distancing themselves from their mothers, most commonly by thinking of them as 'a little old lady, not my Mum'. However, because the content of the caring relationship was very much a mixture of love as well as labour, and of affection as well as obligation, carers more often than not experienced great difficulty in adjusting to a relationship with a mother whose physical and mental condition was deteriorating and with whom a warm emotional relationship often became difficult. Furthermore, because the tensions between mother and daughter were being played out in the private sphere of the home, and because the mother's response not infrequently took the form of failing to co-operate in her care, daughters often found it additionally difficult to look outside the primary caring relationship for help and support.

Carers and kin

Qureshi and Walker's (1986, 1987) research has revealed the existence of a perceived hierarchy of preferred carers, with the daughter being the firm first choice in the absence of a spouse. The majority of our unmarried-daughter carers 'drifted' into caring because both they and their peer groups assumed it was natural for them to do so. Unmarried women of this generation usually assumed they would live in the parental home. There were pragmatic as well as normative reasons for so doing: building societies did not readily give mortgages to unmarried women until the 1970s. Married daughters, on the other hand, were much more likely to have taken a conscious decision to care, and to have come into conflict with siblings over the assumption of primary responsibility for the caring task.

Our data provided considerable evidence of fierce sibling rivalry and bitterness over the caring issue. Three of the twenty only-children carers expressed the unsolicited view that while they had initially wished they had someone else with whom to share the burden of caring, they now felt that the arguments with siblings over who should do what would have been too great. Only one respondent expressed bitterness at being an only child.

For the most part the unmarried-daughter carers with married brothers or sisters (fourteen in all) accepted that they would take primary responsibility for the personal care of their mothers, especially if, as was usually the case, they had continued to live in the parental home. Most, however, looked to siblings for social support of various kinds. Brothers were not expected to give assistance with personal-care tasks, but they were expected to provide financial support if it was necessary and if they were able, and, like sisters, to express some appreciation of the work the carer was doing. Appreciation, whether from kin, neighbours, friends, professionals, or most important of all, from the mother herself, is usually the only 'payment' the carer receives and, in the case of kin, particular bitterness was reserved for siblings who never acknowledged the role played by the carer or sympathized with her difficulties. Respondents were also aware that married brothers were often anxious to protect themselves from demands that they, or more particularly their wives, could not meet.

Non-resident sisters were expected to do rather more and on the whole did so, especially by giving the carer a break. In some cases this was acknowledged to work well, but, as one unmarried carer observed, it could be difficult for the full-time carer to listen to the mother's account of the treats and privileges accorded her on her two week annual visit to another of her children. In some cases this latent tension increased with time, the carer both wanting a break and yet wishing to defend her status as the primary care-giver, caring being for many women a matter of both identity and activity.

Married women experienced direct conflict with their siblings over the provision of personal care. Most struggled to balance caring for their mothers with caring for husbands and children and, as the mother's condition deteriorated, the struggle became increasingly difficult and the conflict between their various responsibilities intensified. They would have welcomed some relief, but, as for the unmarried carers, once the co-resident caring relationship had been established, the part played by other kin tended to be limited and rarely to include anything but sporadic respite care. Even in cases where carers did receive good emotional support, it would be more correct to describe them as being 'helped' rather than as care being 'shared'.

Carers and friends and neighbours

During the early period of co-resident caring, when the carer may have felt it inadvisable to leave her mother for an extended period of time, but when the mother was otherwise mobile and capable of performing many personal care tasks for herself, it was not uncommon for both mother and daughter to have a number of friends and neighbours who 'dropped in' on an occasional or regular basis. We found that this period sometimes lasted for many years before marked deterioration in the mother's condition triggered a significant shift in the nature of the relationship between carer and person cared for, on the one hand, and friends and/or neighbours on the other.

Carers reported that their mothers' social networks shrank rapidly as their physical and/or mental health worsened. As a greater amount of their own time and energy was absorbed by caring, carers became more reliant on friends for emotional support, but, at the same time, found friendships harder to sustain. Those most likely to be maintained were local ones and only to the degree that the friends could cope with the mother's condition. Willmott (1986) has written about the difficulty in differentiating between the role of friend and neighbour and about the importance of recognizing as 'local friends' those who have in previous studies been categorized as neighbours. In the case of one of our respondents, a relationship with a neighbour during two years of full-time care for her mother became a friendship; after the mother's death a rupture took place and the friend reverted to the status of neighbour. Once the mother's mediating influence was removed, the basis for the friendship also disappeared.

On the whole, those categorized by the carer as neighbours tended to give practical support and those as friends emotional support. This may well be for the reason suggested by Allan (1984): because friendship is often based on sociability and enjoyment, it does not necessarily translate into help with caring tasks. On the other hand, although very few carers received any help with personal care tasks from anyone but paid helpers, friends were marginally more likely than neighbours to help in this way. Carers very rarely expressed bitterness about those friends who 'fell away'; those who remained were valued most for the emotional reassurance they were able to offer. They could usually be counted on to take the carer's side and to reinforce the daughter's perception that it was her mother rather than she who was being unreasonable. Friends who, from personal experience, were able to relate to the lifestyle of the carer were additionally valuable for the greater depth of their understanding or for the way in which they could provide information about services and financial benefits.

While neighbours most commonly performed caring tasks other

than those involving personal tending, their role was closely defined, chiefly by the carer's ideas as to what was appropriate. If neighbours performed a caring task regularly, particularly as sitter, some reciprocity was felt to be very important. It is argued that it is partly this psychological need which justifies use of *paid* neighbours to help with caring tasks (Chambers 1986; Davies and Challis 1986). In our sample the carers who received practical support from neighbours usually left a meal for the sitter.

As Willmott (1986) found, neighbours most commonly practise some sort of surveillance. One respondent reported that a neighbour would check on her mother during the day while she was at work. As she observed, because of her mother's dementia, there was considerable self-interest in her neighbour's actions: 'Well you can understand that because . . . neighbours and gas — it was a certain amount of self-interest as well, but I was very glad of that'.

On the whole there was a shared understanding that both friends and neighbours would maintain some distance from the intimate work of personal tending. Friends offered mainly emotional support and neighbours practical support ancilliary to the main personal-tending tasks.

Carers and paid helpers

Unlike kin, friends, and neighbours, paid workers usually helped respondents with some aspect of personal-care tasks. All our respondents said that they would have liked more assistance from paid helpers and a majority experienced considerable difficulty in obtaining the kind of help they wanted. The first difficulty, for a variety of complex reasons, was in seeking help. Second, when help was offered, the carers often found it to be either inappropriate or unsympathetic. Despite the instances of good practice that were described to us the efforts of paid helpers were often perceived as clumsy usurpations rather than useful supplementation of the carer's own efforts. We shall describe the nature of these difficulties from the carer's point of view in more detail.

Carers who expressed difficulty in seeking help felt that to ask for it was, at some level, to admit failure. Having taken on the responsibility to care, they felt that they should 'see it through'. Two reported that they had had difficulty in recognizing that they needed some help in the first place. This might be common at particular points in the caring period. In order to cope, carers tended to set up fairly rigid routines for personal tending that they followed day in, day out. One respondent was told by her general practitioner (GP) to come back to him when she felt she could no longer cope. The lifting gradually became heavier, the bathing more difficult, and her mother incontinent, but she told us that she could not decide when it was that she could not cope. Jones *et al.* (1983) have shown that some 60 per cent of carers experience health problems themselves. This was reflected in our sample, no fewer than nine of our carers experiencing breakdowns after caring ended. The established caring routine may itself mask strain and, because it is performed unquestioningly, make it appear to outsiders that the carer is managing 'to cope'. In the later stages of caring both daughters and mothers tended to become very isolated and the protective web of the caring routines became very difficult for the carers to break, to the long-term detriment of their own health. As Graham (1983) has pointed out, in some circumstances the act of 'coping' can inflict damage on women's health.

Some respondents were too attached to the role of carer to seek help. These included ten women who expressed doubts as to whether strangers, even trained workers, could understand 'the peculiarities of your mum'. Some of them had thought that no one else *could* care properly for their mothers. These carers both took immense pride in the way in which they looked after their mothers and identified wholly with the role of carer. Three other carers would have liked some help but felt that it would be disloyal to their mothers to ask for it. In these cases the mothers were all mentally alert and the daughters feared making them think they were burdensome.

Fourteen respondents felt at some time that they could not cope and were prepared to ask for help, but they too felt that they could not ask, a feeling which often stemmed partly from the carer's sense of guilt and partly from a sense of personal inadequacy. Levin *et al.* (1983) found this to be a major cause of carers' reluctance to seek help. A mother's reluctance to be cared for by others also often played a part in determining a carer's behaviour.

Not only did many carers feel they should not or could not ask for help, but, at a more practical level, they did not know where to turn for advice. 'You're very much on your own, there's no um, I didn't really know where to go I suppose. I would now but I didn't at the time.' One carer who was about to take on the responsibility for caring for another relative remarked: 'Having done all this with mother it doesn't worry me because I know where to go'. Not knowing 'where to go' is one of the most worrying and frustrating aspects of caring. Carers were also frustrated by the variability in services (those who had moved from one area to another were often astonished by this) and by the considerable number of gaps and overlaps in provision. Despite the preponderance of middle-class women in our sample, who were for the most part both well-educated and articulate, most had little expertise in seeking help from official agencies.

Respondents who got over both the hurdle of deciding to seek help and that of finding out where to go for it often met with a lack of either an appropriate or a sympathetic response. One respondent had wanted more domiciliary nursing help but her GP offered only a hospital bed for her mother. Another wanted some respite care each week, but was offered only a fortnight per year. Depending on their extra-caring commitments and interests (including husbands, children, jobs, further education courses), as well as on the health of their mothers, carers' needs were highly individual. The carer who struggled to maintain some element of her extra-caring identity by keeping up her attendance once a week at an adult education course, for example, required help to enable her to succeed and thereby to lessen the strain of caring.

Given the need most carers felt to keep up strict caring routines, it was very important that whatever help was offered be reliable. Meals-on-wheels, bathing attendants, nursing help, and transport to day care were all criticized for unreliability. If carers had hesitated to draw on a service in the first place for fear of upsetting their mothers, a bad experience made it harder to persuade their mothers to accept any alternative form of assistance. Most of the thirteen respondents whose mothers attended day-care centres ended up having to chauffeur their mothers themselves because they were not on the ambulance route or because the timing of the transport did not fit into their work routine.

As important to many carers as the quality of the practical help they sought was the degree of sympathy with which their requests for help or advice were met. A majority agreed that they would have liked, above all, 'someone at the end of a telephone who you didn't feel you'd be a nuisance to' and who could be called on at a moment's notice to advise. Many carers felt that the response they received from paid staff indicated a lack of understanding not just of their immediate needs, but of the broader meaning of caring. GPs in particular came in for a great deal of criticism in this respect. One respondent experienced considerable tension as a result of her efforts to balance looking after her husband and caring for her mother with her determination to preserve her identity and status as an employed person. Her GP's simplistic solution to her problems was neither appropriate nor sympathetic. Another respondent commented: 'Doctors don't know . . . they don't listen . . . and they're *busy.*'

The lack of appreciation on the part of many paid helpers of the meaning of caring for the carer may become acute when the elderly persn is admitted to an institution. Of the thirteen carers whose mothers were in hospitals or nursing homes for more than the last few days of their lives, nine reported feeling guilt and a profound sense of loss. Paid helpers were reported to be more likely to behave as though the carer's problems were now over: she should relax and leave her mother to their care. However, given the fact that many carers felt they knew their mothers' needs best, and given that their sense of self worth was often interwoven with the activity of caring, the adjustment to their mother's institutionalization usually proved difficult.

> I couldn't switch off. I used to go and see her more or less every day. When she first went in she was quite bright, but they said, 'We'd much rather you didn't come in every day because you're going to upset her'.

This respondent also felt that the staff did not look after her mother as well as she had. Finding fault with the treatment given to the loved one may be a way of projecting the anger of grief felt when the person is ill or dying, but it may be also be engendered by an awareness on the part of the carer that her role as carer has been usurped, with no recognition given as to how her role might be modified or gradually phased out.

Conclusions

The research revealed that the matrix of relationships involving both mothers and daughters was often subject to conflict and that it was often difficult for informal care to be effectively shared. In general, the experience of our respondents suggested that the mother/daughter relationship became increasingly difficult over time, and the mother's lack of co-operation in her care could itself constitute a barrier to the daughter seeking help. The carer's extra-caring relationships with kin, friends, and neighbours varied in frequency and quality, and tended to attenuate as the mother's dependency increased. As they did so, the primary relationship between mother and daughter became more intense, and the pair became more isolated. Our respondents had firm ideas as to what help they could get from friends and neighbours: help with the growing burden of personal tending tasks was rarely considered appropriate. Kin were expected to help by providing periodic respite care, but once the co-resident caring relationship had been established, all those close to the carer assumed that the primary responsibility for caring rested with the resident daughter. The 'network of informal social support' (Willmott 1986) seemed to function only before the dependency of the person cared for necessitated the full-time presence of a carer, for example in the often lengthy period during which a daughter felt it unwise to leave her mother overnight, or for the weekend, but when things were otherwise functioning 'normally'. Later, when the mother's condition had deteriorated and the burden of personal tending intensified, the carer was increasingly reliant on paid helpers as a bulwark against strain.

Many carers expressed deep appreciation of particular aspects of the services they received from paid workers, for example of the 'body help' provided by district nurses. However, their perceptions of the shortcomings of paid help and the weight they attached to them are important because of what they reveal about the ways in which help is so rarely carer-centred in its orientation.

Because informal care comprises a mixture of labour and love, and may constitute both identity and activity, it is often difficult successfully to inject paid help. Some of our carers *wanted* help, but still felt that they knew what was best for their mothers; some were at breaking-point and *needed* help, but were unable to ask for it; and some did not seek aid because their mothers refused to contemplate offers of help from outside. From the accounts of caring given to us, it would appear that paid helpers tended to identify a solution to a particular problem without sufficient attention to the carer's perspective, the meaning caring had for her, and her other priorities. The GP who advised a married respondent to give up her job assumed wrongly that her income provided 'pin money' only and failed to appreciate that it was crucial both to paying the mortgage and to her determination to sustain an identity beyond that of carer. In addition, carers often found the services provided unreliable. Informal care is promoted by government and often preferred by elderly people because it provides the most flexible response to their needs. However, our evidence suggests that it involves carers in the construction of fairly rigid caring routines in order to survive. Meeting the needs of their mothers for personal tending required the careful timetabling of feeding, bathing, and toileting. In cases where carers called on paid workers for help in performing such tasks, it was crucial that the support was offered at the time and in the manner considered appropriate by the carer and cared-for person. Thus, if paid workers are successfully to complement the carer's work, it is they who must demonstrate the greatest flexibility of all.

We may conclude that co-resident carers do want help. Informal and formal care should therefore not be regarded as mutually exclusive alternatives. Attempts to 'interweave' them must begin by considering the primary caring relationship of mother and daughter. Such an approach works outwards from an assessment of the nature and quality of that primary caring relationship to the extra-caring relationships of both carer and cared-for person, and finally to ways of supplementing the carer's work. Because relatively little attention has been given to ways of working in delivering care at home, it may be more helpful to return to the early work of Abrams (1978), echoed in the more recent work of Pinker (1985) which has emphasized the differences between formal and informal systems of care, and the importance of respecting those differences. Paid workers serve as the bulwark against strain for informal carers and it is crucial that better ways are found to 'support the supporters'. Our data revealed that much of the help that was offered was unreliable, inappropriate, or unsympathetic. Efforts to 'interweave' care must take more account of the informal carers' perspectives if they are to be effective.

Notes

1. The exploratory nature of the study justified a non-representative sample and in addition to the National Council for Carers and their Elderly Dependents, respondents were located via the Association of Carers, a letter to a local newspaper, a social services department of a London borough, the manager of a Part III home, a hospital carers' group and by personal contact. The pattern of experiences, especially in respect to what we defined as problematic or supportive mother/daughter relationships, did not differ significantly between those who responded directly to a letter or article in a newspaper or carers' newsletter, and those who were indirect referrals, largely from health or social services staff, who had obtained consent in principle from respondents prior to our contacting them.
2. The problems of assessing women's social class have provoked considerable controversy, see for example the exchange in *Sociology* 18 (November 1984).
3. In this chapter we define the term 'paid workers' to include some or all of the variety of professional and trained people who might come into contact with a carer and person-cared-for — for example, statutory workers such as general practitioners, district-nurses, social workers, therapists and home helps, and non-statutory paid workers such as Crossroads care attendants.

References

Abrams, P. (1978) 'Community care: some reseach problems and priorities', in J.A. Barnes and N. Connelly (eds) *Social Care Research*, London: Bedford Square Press.

Allan, G. (1984) 'Friendship and care for elderly people', *Ageing and Society* 6 (1) 1–12.

Audit Commission (1986) *Making a Reality of Community Care*, London: Audit Commission for Local Authorities in England and Wales.

Bayley, M. (1973) *Mental Handicap and Community Care: A Study of Mentally Handicapped People in Sheffield*, London: Routledge & Kegan Paul.

Bulmer, M. (1986) 'Can caring come together?', *New Society* 4 July: 18–20.

Chambers, P. (1986) 'Paid neighbours improve care for frail elderly', *Geriatric Medicine*, November: 42–4.

Cloke, Christopher (1985) *Caring for Carers. A Directory of Initiatives*, Mitcham: Age Concern England Information and Policy Department.

Davies, B. and Challis, D. (1986) *Matching Resources to Needs in Community Care*, Aldershot: Gower.

EOC (1982) *Caring for the Elderly and Handicapped: Community Care Policies and Women's Lives*, Manchester: Equal Opportunities Commission.

Ermisch, John (1983) *The Political Economy of Demographic Change*, London: Heinemann.

Evandrou, M., Arber, S., Dale, A., and Gilbert, G.N. (1986) 'Who cares for elderly? Family care provision and receipt of statutory services', in C. Phillipson, M. Bernard, and P. Strang (eds) *Dependency and Independence in Old Age: Theoretical Perspectives and Policy Alternatives*, London: British Society of Gerontology.

Evers, H. (1985) 'The frail elderly woman: emergent questions in ageing and women's health', in E. Lewin and V. Olesen (eds) *Women, Health and Healing*, London: Tavistock.

Fisher, L.R. (1986) *Linked Lives. Adult Daughters and their Mothers*, New York: Harper and Row.

Graham, Hilary (1983) 'Caring: a labour of love', in Janet Finch and Dulcie Groves (eds) *A Labour of Love: Women, Work and Caring*, London: Routledge & Kegan Paul.

Hadley, R. (1981) 'Social Service Departments and the community', in E.M. Goldberg and S. Hatch (eds) *A New Look at the Personal Social Services*, London: Policy Studies Institute.

Jones, D.A., Victor, C.R., and Vetter, N.J. (1983) 'Carers of the elderly in the community', *Journal of the Royal College of General Practitioners* 33: 707–10.

Leat, D., and Gay, P. (1987) *Paying for Care: A Study of Policy and Practice in Paid Care Schemes*, London: Policy Studies Institute.

Levin, E., Sinclair, I., and Gorbach, P. (1983) *The Supporters of Confused Elderly Persons at Home*, London: National Institute of Social Work.

Matthews, Sarah H. (1979) *The Social World of Old Women*, Beverley Hills: Sage, Library of Social Research No. 78.

Mount, F. (1983) *The Subversive Family*, London: Allen & Unwin.

Parliamentary Paper (1981) DHSS, Secretary of State for Scotland, Northern Ireland and Wales, *Growing Older*, Cmnd. 8173, London: HMSO.

Pinker, R.A. (1985) 'Social policy and social care: divisions of responsibility', in J.A. Yoder, J.M.L. Jonker, and R.A.B. Leaper (eds) *Support Networks in a Caring Community*, Dordrecht: Martinus Nijhoff.

Qureshi, H. and Walker, A. (1986) 'Caring for elderly people: the family and the state'. In C. Phillipson and A. Walker (eds) *Ageing and Social Policy. A Critical Assessment*, Aldershot: Gower.

Qureshi, H. and Walker, A. (1987) *The Caring Relationship*, London: Routledge & Kegan Paul.

Wicks, M. and Henwood, M. (1984) *The Forgotten Army: Family Care and Elderly People*. London: Family Policy Studies Centre.

Willmott, P. (1986) *Social Networks. Informal Care and Public Policy*, Research Report 655, London: Policy Studies Institute.

Chapter eleven

Residential Care and the Maintenance of Social Identity: Negotiating the Transition to Institutional Life

Jennifer Hockey

The context of care

Highfield House was a local authority residential home for elderly people, purpose-built at the periphery of a small town in the North-east of England, within half a mile of one of its neighbouring villages, Moorgate.[1] It accommodated forty-six individuals 'in need of care and attention not otherwise available'.[2] For most it offered a private bed-sitting room in conjunction with communal lounge and dining-room facilities. A staff consisting of matron, care assistants, and care aids was available, should a resident need help in washing, dressing, getting about, or become ill. Given that this institution was the final home of most of its residents, the care of sick and dying people was an intrinsic aspect of its role.

In other words, Highfield House constituted a context within which living and dying went on at close quarters, a state of affairs which was at odds with contemporary culturally specific practices which ensure the maintenance of a marked spatial, social, temporal, and conceptual boundary between life and death. Thus, for example, less than 30 per cent of all deaths in Great Britain now occur in private homes, the domestic space within which individuals have lived.[3] In Highfield House, the potential tension arising out of the anomalous proximity of living and dying was customarily resolved through strategies such as creating a spatial distance between those residents categorized by staff as 'fit' and those categorized as 'frail', or guarding against the sudden appearance of a corpse among living residents by checking the breathing of sleeping residents hourly through the night.[4] 'Life' went on; but deterioration and death, though largely implicit or submerged, were always waiting in the wings.

During my period of anthropological fieldwork in Highfield House (1980–1), most residents were over 75 years old, more than half being over 85 years. Ill or relatively immobile residents, who once would have been accommodated on the home's downstairs, 'frail' corridor, inched their zimmer frames along to bed-sitting rooms on the first floor. Their care involved staff in carrying meal trays and wheelchairs upstairs; and, potentially, carrying a seated corpse downstairs in the home's small lift.

Social identity

It was within this context that residents sought to maintain the social identity developed in the course of their eighty or ninety years of past life. The meaning and the role of the memories, possessions, and personal style remaining to them is the focus of this chapter. The record of their past lives in most cases was available only in their own verbal accounts, but it was also embodied, implicitly, in their possessions and their gestures. Personal identities, therefore, consisted in the selective oral accounts of what had gone before; in those remaining personal belongings through which memories were evoked; in the scars or bodily weaknesses which marked some of a lifetime's formative incidents; and in the gestures and speech patterns through which the institutional present was negotiated. Assigning meaning to these materials required an awareness of the part they played within a death-imbued context.

A guide to that context was offered to prospective residents by the local authority's Social Services Department in the form of a pamphlet. It advised them that, on admission to the home, tenancy or ownership of their own home must be given up; that their furniture could not be accommodated; that the officer-in-charge would take possession of their money, valuables, pension book, and medicines; that the times and places for receiving visitors were circumscribed; that the use of alcohol and tobacco must be moderated. This formal notification of the compulsory shedding of possessions, responsibilities, and personal space not only served to erode aspects of experience constitutive of social identity; in the context of a residential home for elderly people, it also carried the implication that death is the impending reality.

Those people who took on membership of the institutional category, 'resident', became one of a far from homogeneous population. Whilst sharing membership of an age-based social category, 'the elderly', residents differed in age across the thirty or more years from the early sixties to the late nineties. Some residents first met seventy years previously on the long benches of Moorgate village school. Some recognized one another from their former, prominent professional positions within local small town society. For some, Highfield House was the last in a long series of institutions which had accommodated them throughout their lives. Of those who were resident for at least part of my nine-month stay, sixteen needed little special care, ten were reliant upon a zimmer frame, seven had difficulty in communicating, and twelve more could neither communicate nor walk with ease. Some residents had multiple forms of dependency — for example, among those already referred to, three were totally immobile and five were troubled with incontinence. Thus, in terms of age, social status, and degree of frailty, the residents of Highfield House were a markedly disparate population. What they all had in common, however, was the experience of living in the same institutional space, and of having no additional domestic context of their own. Similarly, the requirement that all but the bed-bound should eat together in the dining-room brought constant exposure to deteriorating strangers and therefore a reminder of the imminence of their own deaths. As a result each resident's sense of personal identity was under threat. They shared a severed connection with their past, a present life among individuals whose age, degree of dependency, and social background varied enormously, and an exposure to the idea of death and the process of dying.

To find out how residents managed this threatening set of circumstances I sought answers to three questions. They were, first, what is the significance for residents of their former way of life?; second, how do they make sense of the transition to institutional life?; and third, through what strategies do they maintain their social identity within the home?

Two lives

Material drawn from two tape-recorded life histories, one of an 84 year-old former 'shopgirl', Ethel Carr, one of an 82 year-old former schoolmaster, Arthur Grant, gives an initial insight into residents' perceptions of a former self and its subsequent transitions.[5]

Ethel Carr had been born in the local town in 1896. Having served an apprenticeship in the confectionery trade, she was set up by her mother in a small business near the town centre. Like about a quarter of the female residents, Ethel had no children and, unmarried, she worked on in her shop for more than forty years, supporting her parents in their old age. Ethel and I had lived a few streets from one another, albeit not simultaneously, and her recorded life history took off from points of shared knowledge — local people, shops, doctors' surgeries — into an assemblage of snapshot incidents spanning the previous sixty years.

The following extract from the record exemplifies the mix of broad appraisal and highly specific incident which characterized the form of Ethel's reminiscence. It sheds light on the first question, concerning residents' perceptions of a former way of life. She told me:

Ah, but you know, people were different in them days to what they are now. It was true friendship and true neighbourhood, you know. They were very friendly, helped a lot. Oh, I never need want a thing.

I just need ask, you know. Used to open the shop door and shout. One woman said to me, 'Do you want anything down the street?' I says, 'Well, bring me two kippers'. I like kippers for me tea. They used to be very cheap in them days. Anytime she passed, doesn't matter if the shop was full, she used to shout, 'Do you want any kippers, Miss Carr?' I used to say, 'Do you think I live on kippers!' By, its a different life now, isn't it, not the same. Because I was young then, you know, and energetic. See, the College boys all used to come. They couldn't get anything at College in them days. And they used to come 'bout ten o'clock and I used to make little buns and fill them with cream, and sell them for a penny. And I used to make, perhaps, four, you know, trays of those. They called my shop 'the Bun Shop' at the College. Its mixed now, isn't it, girls and boys. Eh, yes.

Ethel's clear sense of herself within the context of 'them days' can be set alongside the powerfully recalled account which Arthur Grant, former schoolmaster, gives of himself during adolescence. Born in 1898, one of the five children of a mining family in Moorgate village, Arthur grew up within the rigid framework of the United Methodist Chapel. 'That was our life — chapel', he told me;

But at weekends, Saturdays, we were real toffs — when we grew up to about sixteen, seventeen. Real toffs. If you weren't playing football for the football team, get our best suit, walking cane, walking stick, white gloves and kid gloves. Posh. Down to town. Market-place. Spend all afternoon and part of the night there. 'Course the market-place was full then, of stalls, you know. Big-band show, like. Randolph Williams's big organ used to take up the whole part of the place and play marches. There were quack doctors there and all sorts of things, pulling teeth out and selling patent medicines and all sorts of things. The place was packed besides the closed-in market where you could go at any time. The whole square was filled up. So we had to go down there every Saturday, or down on to the racecourse for a cricket match or something like that. We were always poshed up. All went together. Real lads. Cane, straw benchers. One-and-sixpence for a straw hat with a green band on, two-and-sixpence for a bigger one, very hard, a cord round the back to fasten on to your lapel here with a button so the wind wouldn't blow it away. We thought we were the bees' knees then. Striding away down to town there, walking of course. Walking-sticks, some had chamois gloves, you know, some patent leather ones. All had walking-sticks. One or two had spats. We thought we were something.

In the case of both Ethel and Arthur, a former self survived in vivid snapshots of energy, youth, and self-importance — 'real toffs', 'young then, you know, and energetic', 'the bees' knees'.

With regard to the second question, concerning the transition to institutional life, both these residents had found it to be a period of demanding change and loss. How they each understood and made sense of their losses was, however, rather different. In both cases, critical events which had taken place in late adolescence, in the years around 1915, were seen to be influential with respect to their circumstances in 1981. References to these events were offered readily. Rather than the outcome of any prompting on my part, speculation and appraisal were their primary preoccupations, as well as those of many other residents.

Ethel Carr identified the personal relationship with her mother as crucial to the life course she was to follow. 'Mothers shape their daughters' destinies', she said, going on to describe her mother's 'narrowness', her refusal to admit potential marriage partners, even friends to the family home. After a harsh apprenticeship in a town some twenty miles away — where she was woken with a thrown apple at 5 a.m. and worked until breakfast at 8 a.m. — Ethel began business life at the age of twenty. 'Oh, I was too young. My mother put me in and I had to bake and manage all the business. I had no youth, I had no youth. Because, I mean, I had to work practically night and day.' Ethel said: 'It's hard, a life on your own. You take a lot of knocks. People think there's a lot of things you don't know about, not having been married'.

It was during this same period that Arthur Grant finished his very successful education at a prestigious local school. Rather than a personal relationship, it was a world event, the Great War, which Arthur saw as crucial to all that followed. He told me:

I was called up straight away. After that — *fini*. No more fiddling [violin playing]. Two-and-a-half years in Italy. Made a wreck of me. Came back with nothing, not a halfpenny, no money. I applied for college, of course, and credentials were alright. I managed to get in, on the understanding that I passed the doctor, coming straight from the war. If he had failed me I don't know what I would have done. So I persuaded him to let me, I pleaded with him. I'd been wounded slightly, but it was malaria and poison gas. I knew what was wrong. I said, 'Give me a chance, man.' I said, 'I can last two years of this, after two-and-a-half years of that.' He says, 'Alright, Mr Grant. Ten and six, please.'

Of his present health and circumstances, Arthur said:

I'm getting weaker every day. I mean, this gas comes back every now and again and malaria — warm days — hits me now and again.

So I just come in here (his bed-sitting room), and wait 'til it oozes out. Say nothing. I don't even bother telling the matron. I get through. I know what to do. You know yourself. You know what to do. But its very noticeable now that the three of us in here that were in the First War — there's George, big Jimmy, and meself — all our legs, they're going. Sometimes we can't walk. They're afflicted in the same way.

Nobody would believe it, nobody would believe it. We're suffering for it now, but there we are. It comes back now and again. I don't wake up screaming or anything like that, you know, it doesn't affect me in that way at all. But I know when the malaria comes back and I know when the gas comes back. Feel rotten. Just have to square up to it, that's all. Frostbite. All for sixpence a day.

In Ethel's case, admission to residential care came after a period of thirteen years spent living in local sheltered accommodation for elderly people. She understood her admission to be on account of 'bad arthritis' in her hands which, temporarily, left her unable to lift a cup. Of the transition to institutional care, she said, 'Dr Unstone put me in here. I rue the day I came in here.' She told me that she'd only intended to stay in the home for one month and had cried for a week when she first arrived. Time had dragged on and on and now she was resigned — 'I won't live much longer. I'm eighty-four. All my friends are dead' — but resistant:

You lose your independence when you come to these places. I've never had a mistress, you see, I've never had a boss. I'll never be happy here, but I'll have to stick it, 'cos I won't live that long, much longer.

And the money they take off you — hundreds of pounds just for a few weeks. Of course they'll bury me and everything. I'm all on my own, so I have no worries on that score. You never think about old age, do you, you never think. You ought to prepare for it.

In common with a number of other residents, Arthur had been admitted to care after a major operation which, it was decided, left him unfit to continue living alone. Widowed for forty years, he had been living with a brother, the two of them looked after by a housekeeper. He said:

Oh yes, we had a real good time. Then of course, both of us having the operations and his mind went. That was it. He died nearly two years ago. Couldn't carry on meself, not in the house by meself. Housekeeper was a bit older than we were and she retired. There was just the pair of us left, except for me little sister. I did all the housework, painting, decorating, all the lot. Too much. However, I'm not grumbling.

So me son brought me to live with him. 'Course being daft, I had to take ill as well. I had an operation meself and they had me into here. Stirred me up a little bit, she [the Matron] did, she cured me. That's the way it goes. I'm not grumbling.

Arthur's repeated verbal commitment to 'not grumbling' revealed a more resigned stoicism than was evident in Ethel's account. Though hindsight had lead Arthur to the opinion that his chapel upbringing had been 'strict, very strict, too strict', he retained faith in the value of discipline in schools — 'the kids thrived on it'. Acceptance and stoicism were evident when he offered the view that: 'You never know how things change in the world. Where you get to. How things link up, or break up. That's life, you take it as it comes. Sometimes its good, sometimes bad.'

Material from Ethel and Arthur's life-histories spotlighted some shared aspects of the lives of many residents — for example, the transformative role of the First World War for male residents; women's unquestioning commitment to caring for elderly parents; the management of hardship through both stoicism and determined independence; pride in former roles and statuses; bitterness over losses by then forever irredeemable. These two life histories also indicated that, depending on gender, residents perceived and experienced the past and its relationship to the present somewhat differently, and this was confirmed by information from other residents of Highfield House. Gender was also of significance in issues raised by the third question, concerning strategies through which social identity was maintained or negotiated within the residential home.

Gender and the experience of admission

While the home accommodated forty-six residents, almost three-quarters of them were women. Of the twelve men who lived in Highfield House during my stay, three allowed me to tape their conversation with me. While many of the women spoke freely about their past lives, only two, when asked, were willing to speak in what they saw as the formal setting of a taped conversation. The discrepancy between women's and men's willingness to give a single, extensive account of their past life was echoed in the style and content of what was said — both on tape and in more informal conversation. In particular, men's chronologically ordered accounts of former roles and the positions they held contrasted with women's vivid and more fragmented asides which described dramatic events from the past or humourous personal interchanges.

It is revealing to look, briefly, at all twelve of the home's male residents. Two of them had spent long periods in institutional care of some kind and remained very much on the fringes of life in Highfield House. Three were frail and/or confused, speaking very rarely and with little coherence. One shared a double bed-sitting room in the home with his more outgoing wife and spoke only rarely himself. Of the other six, five were prominent within the home, among them the three willing for their life histories to be taped. Together, that minority of five male residents who were free from extensive handicap or disability represented a strong, articulate presence within the home.

Arthur Grant offered his life history in a lucid, linear form which began by tracing the passage from school-days shared with three of the home's other residents; included reference to the predominance of chapel and music practice in his early life; and went on to his wartime experience, his teaching career, his retirement, and his children and grandchildren's careers — 'They're all BAs except me. All comfortably well off there, now. No worries. And that's the story.' Details of Arthur's social life, his courting days, and his marriage were given only in response to my further questioning.

Like Arthur Grant, George Smith too had been born in 1898, into a large mining family in Westgate village. As in Arthur's case, Methodism had provided the framework for George's early life, one within which he had remained throughout his life. 'During the whole of my married life I was in the Methodist Church. Now everything that took place, I was always active in it. Nearly every event or position, I was in it.' This sentence, 'every position I was in it', provided the starting-point for the whole of George's life history as he chose to present it — a detailed list of a lifetime's significant roles and achievements. George's oral record is complemented by three local history books he has written and an album of his certificates and photos made by a nephew. In his 'secret drawer' (a locked drawer built into every residents' wardrobe), George kept a little cardboard box containing a British Legion medal and a Christian Endeavour badge. They were to be passed down to his nephew when he died.

Albert Lyons was another of the five prominent male residents, older than George and Arthur, approaching his ninetieth birthday. He entered Highfield House with his wife, living on there alone after her death. He spoke freely at all times, his conversation consisting almost entirely of the stories which go to make up his life history. Like George, Albert complemented his tales with scrap-books of photos and press clippings. On tape, it was his career as plumber, joiner, and concert party entertainer; his father's career at the colliery; and his grandfather's career as agricultural engineer and night-watchman, which provided a framework for the story. In addition to scrap-books, still noticeable consequences of industrial injuries to Albert's eyes and feet provided prompts for the re-telling of dramatic incidents from his working life. He also used my tape-recorder to re-create his former role as concert party entertainer, painstakingly retrieving half-forgotten monologues and music hall songs.

208

The ease with which men offered accounts of public roles and positions as life history contrasted with the richness and diversity of women's references to the past. Evers'[6] discussion of the different meanings of institutional care for women and men sheds light on this contrast. She argues that while the identity of retired men rests on the honourable performance of their past employment, women's identity continues throughout life to arise out of the quality of care which they provide within the home — 'A woman's work is never done.'

The shift into institutional care therefore had different implications depending on the resident's gender. Most of the women found themselves bereft of their identity as domestic carer. The men not only experienced continuity in receiving care from women; they also discovered new scope for public 'role-playing' once they moved out of a more private form of domestic life. Thus, for Arthur Grant, George Smith, Jack McIntyre, and Albert Lyons, the public sphere of a residential 'home' represented a context where an acceptable male dependence on female care could quite appropriately go hand in hand with public reference to and re-creation of their former professional or quasi-professional roles. Jack McIntyre, prominent as the residents' male representative on the Friends of Highfield House committee,[7] was aware of the fusion of domestic and public worlds within the home. 'In your own home', he told me, 'you arrange your social life outside, but here you do it all in the same place, on the job.'

What, then, were the important reference points for these elderly men engaged in managing the transition to residential care? Albert Lyons' wife had died after they both had moved into the home. He often told me how she had been taken away from Highfield House for hospital treatment, how he had seen her funeral cortège pass by the home, but was too unwell to attend. In referring frequently to his bereavement Albert was an exception, in that the other men had been admitted after a long period of widowerhood. For them, dependence on female carers, unrelated to them, was acceptable, while the loss of an active role within the outside world was still felt. Within the home, it was therefore through reference to, and re-creation of, the public roles of that outside world that they sought to maintain their social identity.

How did the implications of admission to care and the way in which they responded to it differ for women? Like Arthur Grant, Ethel Carr's personal history is an account of a working life outside the home. However, as in the extract presented earlier, it was told through a mosaic of interchanges with neighbours, shop-girls, customers, and family — and not as a linear progression from school-days through to retirement. On admission to residential care, Ethel had burnt most of her photos taken in and around the shop. Prominent among the remaining few was one which marked a lost personal relationship. Kept on her bedside locker, the photo showed one of her sisters, a former hospital matron. Ethel told me:

> She was at Edinburgh Royal. She went when she was eighteen and she died at 62, and she was at that Edinburgh Royal all those years. She was a real sport, she was short and very fat. I think an awful lot of her. I don't think so much of the other one. But I was upset when she died. She died at 62, and she'd been in hospital life all that time. And when she died they found her dead in bed. She had heart, well she was so fat, you know, little and fat, and liked her food — big, fat rosy face, you know, jolly. They found her dead in bed, in the hospital. And the secretary wrote and said that she had spent her life looking after other people but at the last she needed no-one. Wasn't it lovely put? She died suddenly. Yes, I was sorry about her. I often think about her, poor girl.

Small personal possessions, photos, table napkins and jewellery were the prompts which repeatedly brought such memories to the surface of the women's minds. By contrast, the men's rooms were often strikingly bare, containing little from which details of their tenant's identity might be detected. While men were willing, at a single sitting, to offer a lengthy account of themselves, women, involved in the continuous handling and re-arranging of remnants of a lost domestic context, gave evidence of their pasts in vivid, fleeting asides, which were repeated on many occasions.

For example, one of the institution's daily routines evoked a highly specific personal memory for 92 year-old Grace Heslop. Highfield House took responsibility for all residents' personal washing, and staff frequently returned small piles of ironed laundry to their rooms. When I handed Grace her clean napkin and handkerchief she was prompted to give me an account of her early married life. The damask napkin, labelled with the former couple's initials, was a remnant of the table linen she received at her wedding in 1916. She had been engaged for only a month in 1914 when her fiance, later husband, left to fight in France. He survived The First World War only to be killed in the Second, leaving her with a teenage daughter and a seven year-old son. Two figures which were repeated often, and usually together, by Grace were her age, 92 years, and the length of her widowhood, forty four years. Her account of an incident in her long distant married life was prompted by an emotive coincidence of the time of year and the handling of the napkin. The 9 November, the previous Sunday, had been Armistice Day. 'You get over it', she said, 'its just these times that bring it back.' For Arthur Grant, war had meant a threat to his career and, now, a physical vulnerability. For Grace Heslop, war meant a lost relationship, one which otherwise might have sustained her throughout old age.

Whichever article of personal memorabilia evoked emotion and reminiscence, for women it was often a bereavement or an illness which came readily to mind. Very often these experiences bore a particular relevance to the institutional present and to the quality of the resident's old age. Recurrent themes were the deaths of children in their sixties and seventies; the loss of younger children who might otherwise have cared for a resident in old age; or, very commonly, the death of a male partner who had provided a lifetime's social, emotional, and financial support. Now, as a resident's body became demandingly weaker, that source of comfort was no longer available to them. Thus, for example, Mabel Carey's mention of her husband's recent death, precipitated by my comment on her snake ring (worn by him through two world wars) was rapidly followed by a description of her son's much earlier but most horrific death by drowning in a cesspit in India.

Mabel's friend, Hannah Archer, also a resident, had had eight children by her now dead husband. Her story of a lively family life led her back repeatedly to Vera, her quiet and clinging daughter who had died in her forties from heart trouble. Hannah had overridden Vera's pleas not to be admitted to hospital and it was there that she died within a few hours.

In these examples it was the dead rather than the surviving child or sibling who absorbed the attention, or whose photo was framed on the locker. In the opening remarks they made to me, the women often referred to an earlier bereavement of this kind. Framed within a present of accumulating losses, these deaths were sources of emotional pain which lay very close to the surface. As noted, admission to care brings an additional loss for women in that they leave behind their role as domestic carer. Those who had no-one to survive them lacked any form of personal connectedness with the future, as well as present links with the outside world. Like Ethel Carr, who had burnt all her photos prior to admission, other women had given away their lifetime's possessions. Indeed, Sally Wilkinson, who lacked a family, often referred in rather incoherent speech to her plan to leave her beautiful opal ring to the home's Matron.

The changed significance of earlier bereavements was made explicit by a resident, Annie Crosby. She told me: 'I had a stillborn boy, you see, and I had a terrible do . . . a complete hysterectomy. And of course when I was younger I didn't feel it so much but now I've no-one to care for me.' Similarly, a reference to the death of a male partner was often the starting-point for an appraisal of the circumstances which led to a female resident's admission. When I went into 91 year-old Mrs Porter's room, for example, she showed me her husband's photo on the dressing-table and said, 'he was the best husband in the world'. She began to cry and told me there had been an accident four years previously; he had been sent to a nearby hospital and she had come to Highfield House.

He had died in hospital and she had stayed on in the home 'to sort myself out', 'get myself pulled together'. She had 'vowed' she would not stay when she first came in, but she found everyone so kind that she stayed on to see how things went. She knew her house in the centre of town was too big for her. Eventually, she made up her mind to stay. She said it was important to accept the rules and regulations of the home. There had to be someone at the top and what they said had to go. She had been in charge of a local sweet factory and knew that this was how it had to be. She said a lot of residents grumbled and complained when they had no cause to. She talked a little about the local town, what a close-knit, friendly town it was. She said she had never been back since her admission four years previously — she was 'too much of a coward'.

Many other female residents echoed Mrs Porter's slow acceptance of the inevitability of residential care and, like her, attempted to make the best of it. After Alice Johnson's husband had died she had little alternative but to accept admission to the home, since her daughter was already preoccupied with care of Alice's son-in-law who had suffered a heart attack. She had 'broken her heart' coming into the home, but had got used to it and settled down. She had been there for two years. Most of her family lived just around the corner in Moorgate village.

Janey Firth had had two strokes and eventually became bed-ridden at one of her daughters' homes. The general practitioner had tried repeatedly to persuade her to go into a home. She had refused but after the second stroke she 'studied and studied' and decided she would be better off in a home. She was totally dependent on her daughter and would never get back to her own place. She said: 'You're well fed here, very comfortable. But its not like your own home.' Childlessness, the death of children and the death of a partner were not the only recurrent themes voiced by the home's elderly women as explanations for their present situation. Breakdown in health was another. Janey's perception of her second stroke as having a determining role in her subsequent admission to care was echoed by other women who identified one specific breakdown of health as crucial to the move into care. Lily Armstrong, for example, seldom allowed a day to pass without mention of the doctor who 'tried out' a powerful drug on her, causing her to black-out in the street. At 92, Lily had lived alone and, though she continued to play bowls for her city up to this point, the injuries resulting from her collapse led rapidly to her permanent admission to Highfield House. Similarly Nellie Baldwin told me:

> I fell off a bus was the thing — I never claimed for it. It was a foggy day, foggy night, on the bus — somebody got off and I started to follow them. . . . I could have complained because the conductor wasn't on the lower deck. A fall brings anything on.

Self-Sustaining Strategies

The material presented thus far indicates those areas of past life to which the residents referred most frequently and most readily. Much of it was offered in fleeting conversations as I cleaned residents' sinks, returned their clean laundry, or helped them into the bath. It was not the outcome of structured interviewing but of a spontaneity which suggested that it reflected issues wich constitute a private undercurrent to residents' daily lives.

An institutional present can thus be conceptualized as a framework or grid through which the past is viewed, some of its aspects taking on new, pressing meanings, others fading into insignificance. On the evidence, men's former careers or positions assumed a new significance for them in the diminished 'public' space of Highfield House. For women, specific illnesses and the loss of significant supportive relationships provided a way of making sense of their transition from care-giving to dependence on the care of other women.

These points can be explored more fully by examining the details of daily interactions between residents within the home. Social identity was not only achieved and maintained by re-creation from salient fragments of the past; it was also tested out and if necessary modified continuously in day-to-day experience.

The context for the continuous endeavour was, as noted, the confined space of the home, shared, with a far from homogeneous population, where living and dying went on at close quarters. The assertion of personal identity and the creation of space between the self and undesirable others were implicit, interrelated objectives which under-pinned much that took place. Framed in a fairly immediate sense by the frequent occurrence of death, these objectives reflected not just a sustained comitment to the past, but also an urgent shielding of the self from the prospect of deterioration, of which the presence of other, 'frailer' residents constituted a constant reminder.

Sissy Crowther, a childless widow in her eighties, had come to Highfield House after an unsuccessful attempt to live with a nephew and his wife. She referred to her admission as a personal decision to try to be 'independent' and 'make my home' in the institution. Eight months later she found herself both physically and socially very vulnerable. She shared her bed-sitting room with Ada Brown, a sixty-two year-old mentally handicapped woman. Things went badly between them. Sissy told me: 'Do you know I pay £86 per week to stay here. And I have to share a room with *her*!' She found Ada a great nuisance, as the latter would come in during the afternoon, when she was asleep on the bed, and put her radio on loudly. She also put it on loudly at 6.30 a.m. Staff told her off but Ada insisted she had the Matron's permission. Mrs

Crowther went on to say that Ada had once walked into the room saying: 'Have you got that bloody heater on again!' Mrs Crowther said:

> Well, I'm not used to that sort of thing. Language like that. I don't know what my nephews and nieces would say if they knew. Well, I wouldn't *tell* them. Of course I tend to give in to her which doesn't help. She is a bit simple, you know.

In the dining-room, residents were given, and retained, the same seat for every meal. Sissy Crowther asked to be moved into an alcove seat at the far end of the room. She said she preferred it. 'I can be away from . . . people, here.' She felt she had come into the home too soon. She should have waited another two years. It was not only the social but also the bodily implications of contact with other residents which Sissy began to find oppressive.

As I re-arranged the blanket box and commode she had brought into Highfield House from her home, Sissy told me how helpless she felt. Every day it got worse. She had been in the home for eight months and she felt she had deteriorated enormously in that time. Although she knew she was old, she had never expected this kind of deterioration. Some people had been in seven, eight, or even eleven years, she said, and it did not give her much to look forward to. She was not happy there, she would just have to *make* herself happy.

Sissy managed the oppressiveness of her environment by withdrawing into the dining-room alcove and by refusing to speak to her roommate, Ada. She also drew on her former identity, as a voluntary worker, decorated for organizing canteen services during the last war. Despite increasing mobility problems, she took on the role of visitor to the more genteel but sick residents. After asserting that she would *make* herself happy, she appeared minutes later in the bed-sitting room of another resident, Elsie Hall, where I was cleaning the sink. In field notes, I made the following observation:

Elsie was in bed, curtains drawn, looking and feeling very unwell. Sissy came in to 'visit' and played the sensitive, caring, middle-class sick visitor to perfection. It was an impressive effort on Sissy's part. Elsie Hall was very pleased to be visited and rose to the occasion with a great show of emotion and pained feebleness.

My initial sense that Sissy's visit to Elsie was far from a casual 'dropping-in' was borne out in the frequency with which other female residents took opportunities to move into a caring role. Bereft of most domestic tasks, they were nonetheless surrounded by 'frail' residents who provided scope for expressing the identity of informal carer. So great was the choice of potential recipients that telling discriminations were often made.

Ethel Carr told me that a very confused resident, Alice Hepple, had begun to call for her all the time. Drawing on the metaphor of parental obligation, Ethel avoided the commitment, saying: 'Alice's not one of *mine*! Gran Robson is a different case. I could adopt her. She's such a character' — and indeed, Gran Robson was strong-minded and alert, if a little unsteady on her feet. In discriminating between the two, Ethel knowingly withdrew from contact with the very confused resident. She was aware that she would not only have little success as her carer, but in failing would risk acquiring a similarly undesirable identity. Hence the double meaning of 'Alice's not one of mine.' Ethel disclaimed not only responsibility but also the possible imputation of some shared origin. By contrast, through leading Gran Robson from lounge to dining-room or on walks in the grounds, Ethel was able to identify herself publicly as an able, kindly carer.

Her visibility in this informal role can be set alongside the public positions which male residents took up within the home. Rather than the outcome of personal negotiation, Arthur Grant, Jack McIntrye, Albert Lyons, and George Smith all accepted roles prescribed by the institution itself. Arthur sold newspapers in the dining-room each morning, for example, and directed the residents' rehearsal of a song he had set to music.[8] George Smith propagated cuttings from his plants and sold them to raise funds for the home at open days. Though this project had been shared with a female resident, Grace Heslop, she told me that her contribution had not been acknowledged when the final sum was publicly announced. Albert Lyons kept a pile of cards and a list of all residents' birthdays in his room. Dutifully he sent them out on behalf of the other residents, a formal rather than a personal gesture. His choice of card was often inappropriate as he now had difficulty linking names and faces. When an elderly person died in the home, Jack McIntyre would attend their funeral as the residents' official representative. He also made the public announcements in the dining-room whenever a rehearsal of Arthur's song was due to take place.

Some conclusions

This chapter has explored the issue of social identity for the residents of an old people's home. To this end three questions were raised — the nature of past memories, the rupture with the past at admission, and the negotiation of identity within the institutional present. Through continuous informal contact with residents I became aware that these questions reflected the areas to which residents gave extended thought and often vigorous energy. ·

Residential homes for elderly people are culturally anomalous in that they are confined spaces where living and dying go on at close quarters, where life merges very gradually into death. Within the wider society, culturally specific practices ensure the maintenance of clear boundaries between these two states. Though a home's staff and residents may seek to maintain similar boundaries, in it death remains an ever-present if carefuly muted reality. In addition, the move into such a context involves taking on permanent membership of a purely age-based social category. This form of social organization characterizes all residential homes where elderly people are given terminal care. Here, its implications have been explored through an in-depth study of one particular home.

What aspects of their past and present lives elderly people chose to talk about in this context was an important starting-point in understanding how they had experienced the transition to care. Life histories showed positive images of a former self being vividly recalled as lively reference points within a less glowing present. It was also evident that the question of how such a present had occurred was pressing. Residents traced links between the events of a long distant past, more recent bereavements, and breakdowns in health, and their current life in residential care. Personal qualities, such as stoicism or determined independence, developed throughout a long lifetime, were invoked as still dependable strategies for survival.

Though women and men entered the same institutional context, its implications differed depending on gender. For women, their lifelong commitment to providing domestic care and emotional support within key personal relationships was robbed of a focus. Memory drew them back to those individuals who had once been the recipients of care; fellow residents were perceived as a possible source of substitutes whose presence might provide a way of re-creating an earlier role. By contrast the men, who made up just one-quarter of the home's populaton, drew on an identity arising out of their public working-life. This was apparent in their recorded life histories, and exemplified out in their willingness to take on public roles within the home.

The study shows that for the residents of Highfield House a stable sense of identity was critical; it was sought determinedly through reminiscence, and was manifest in interpersonal interaction. Whatever policies with respect to the way death is managed may be adopted by the staff of residential homes, and however well the residents of homes may know each other as lifelong members of the same local community, the anomalous proximity of life and death, and the different losses sustained by women and by men are likely to be inevitable features of residential homes for elderly people in our society. The responses of the residents of Highfield House give us revealing insights into the quality of experience encountered by those destined eventually to enter such an institution.

Notes

1. To ensure confidentiality, all proper names, as well as the name of the home, have been changed.
2. The National Assistance Act, 1948, Pt. III, Section 21, requires that residential care shall be provided 'for those in need of care and attention not otherwise available'.
3. *Annual Abstract of Statistics*, No. 120, 1984 edition, London: HMSO.
4. J. Hockey (1985) 'Cultural and social interpretations of 'dying' and 'death' in a residential home for elderly people in the North East of England', *Curare*, Sonderband 4. (Sterben und Tod. Verhandlungen der 7. Int. Fachkonferenz Ethnomedizin. 5/8-4-84).
5. Life history tapes constituted one form of field material recorded when residents offered particularly extensive and detailed accounts of past lives. Participant-observation in my role of care aid was the primary research method.
6. H. Evers (1981) 'Care or custody? The experiences of women patients in long-stay geriatric wards', in B. Hutter and G. Williams (eds) *Controlling Women*, London: Croom Helm.
7. The Friends of Highfield House were a group of middle-aged women and men who raised funds and organized social activities for the residents.
8. J. Hockey (1983) 'Just a song at twilight. Resident's coping strategies expressed in musical form', in D. Jerrome (ed.) *Ageing in Modern Society*, London: Croom Helm.

© Jennifer Hockey

Chapter twelve

Bridging the Gap Between Hospital and Home: Two Models of Discharge Care for Elderly People[1]

Jill Russell and Maria Brenton

In this chapter we explore strategies of care and support for elderly people on discharge fron hospital. The ideas arose from work conducted as part of an evaluation of a hospital discharge service in South Glamorgan, one of a growing number of intensive support schemes run, for the most part, as 'pilot schemes', by voluntary organizations (see Russell 1986). Such schemes may be directly linked with their predecessors thirty years ago, again provided by the voluntary sector — the experimental rest homes for elderly people.

Both these models of care strategy originated in response to identified needs of elderly people in the transition period between being in hospital and being considered well enough for self-care at home. It is instructive to ask why each type of scheme arose in the first instance, why the older one appears to have sunk without trace, and what both models tell us about the capability of the mainstream systems of health and social services in providing hospital after-care in this critical period in an elderly person's life. Asking such questions leads us to see how hospital discharge of an elderly person is a key test of the integratedness or otherwise of welfare support. What is perhaps most interesting from a policy perspective is to ask why over a thirty-year timespan, there has been no 'system learning' — why it is that a seemingly enduring and evident need has provoked little in the way of mainstream system change and is still being addressed by temporary measures 'tacked on' to the statutory services from the voluntary sector.

In this chapter, therefore, we compare these two forms of post-discharge, short-term provision, as a way of exploring why the needs of elderly people on discharge from hospital have remained at the periphery of state welfare policies for them. Our tentative conclusions concern the institutional and professional rigidities of health and social services, the low social and professional esteem in which elderly people are held, and the reluctance of policy-makers to confront system defects and professional boundaries in the interests of a vulnerable group of people who do not neatly fit pre-ordained system categories. The marginal and ambiguous status of convalescence as a medical construct is also briefly explored, in a discussion of the definition, construction, and de-construction by policy-makers of 'need' among elderly people.

Rest homes for the elderly

'Experimental' rest homes were established in the 1950s as an institutional response to the problem of giving care and support to the elderly on discharge from hospital (Adams 1954; Dickson 1978; Means and Smith 1985). Geriatric medicine was then in its infancy, raising the expectation that elderly people in hospital could be rehabilitated and regain their independence (see Bosanquet 1978). The National Assistance Act of 1948 was also new, with domiciliary services still poorly developed. The Act obliged local authorities to provide *accommodation* for elderly people in need, but this was defined as being only for the healthy old, and not for the placement of the frail elderly leaving hospital (Means and Smith 1985). Domiciliary services were seen as largely the responsibility of the voluntary sector and did not become mandatory upon local authorities until much later (Townsend 1981).

The concept of the rest home was derived from the belief that a gap existed between the accommodation provided by the welfare authority and that provided by the hospitals (Dickson 1978). The National Corporation for the Care of Old People (NCCOP) (one of the key voluntary organizations involved in the provision of rest homes) argued that there was in practice 'a gap between the Acts (National Health Service and National Assistance), and it is the Corporation's intention to place these Rest Homes, as it were, across the gap' (quoted in Means and Smith 1985: 184) The provision of rest homes was seen as lessening 'the liability to premature breakdown and readmission to hospital . . . by the gradual transition . . . from hospital to home conditions, and time [being] given to ensure proper resettlement' (Adams 1954: 488). Part of the function of the rest home was 'to give patients a chance to adjust themselves to change while still under supervision', before returning to their own homes (ibid.: 487).

The concept of the rest home was also inextricably bound to orthodox medical thinking about the nature and value of convalescence that prevailed at the time. The subject of convalescence is a fascinating one that has been little researched. During the first half of the twentieth century, a short stay in a convalescent home after a period in hospital was considered a routine and even necessary part of medical treatment (Ministry of Health 1959). This traditional convalescence was defined by a Ministry of Health report on the subject as consisting of 'rest, good food and fresh air with medical oversight available and a minimum of nursing care, in as pleasant surroundings as possible' (ibid.). The same report explained how, 'since these necessities were in the past not normally available in the patient's home, they came to be specially provided by a system of convalescent homes'. By the 1950s, however, 'passive' or 'classical' convalescence was beginning to be regarded by the medical profession as an optional luxury; in the words of one doctor — as 'a pleasant convenience to the patient or a thoughtful gesture by the referring physician' (ibid). The general improvement in the nation's health and the improvement in home conditions were given as reasons for this changing view. In addition, the medical emphasis, following the acute stage of a patient's illness, was increasingly on the value of active rehabilitation in recovery units of hospitals or hospital annexes.

In the early days of the National Health Service there existed, within and outside it, a confusing array of recuperative holiday homes, convalescent homes, pre-convalescent beds and recovery units, hospitals, and homes (Drain 1957). The admissions policies of these institutions tended to discriminate against elderly people, on the grounds that they would be difficult to discharge, thus eroding the essentially short-term nature of the residential provision (King Edward's Hospital Fund 1954; Ministry of Health 1959). When rest homes were established, they were presented as special recovery homes for the elderly, although Means and Smith, in their study of the development of welfare services for the elderly, suggest that in practice they 'differed very little from an ordinary convalescent home run by the hospital authorities' (Means and Smith 1985: 185). In their fourteenth annual report, the NCCOP stated that 'by and large these [rest] Homes provide a period of what might loosely be called convalescence which enables many patients to recover some of their former activity and regain confidence in themselves' (NCCOP 1961).

Means and Smith decribe how, in 1950-1, the trustees of the King Edward's Hospital Fund for London set aside £250,000 to establish a series of 23–35 bed rest homes in London to be administered by the Regional Hospital Boards, but run by voluntary organizations. The NCCOP also established four such homes. In principle, these homes had more of an inter-sectoral identity in that the financial arrangements were that patients should be supported by either the hospital or the welfare authorities. This operated by screening patients and, in Dickson's words, 'designating them as either a welfare or hospital responsibility depending upon the degree of their rehabilitation' (Dickson 1978). The NCCOP hoped that one of the spin-offs of this system would be greater co-operation between the health and welfare services; indeed, they saw joint working as one of the key innovative features of the experimental homes. A review of the NCCOP homes stated that they offered 'an opportunity for the different authorities to come together on a common ground to iron out their difficulties with individual cases and to encourage them to work more closely in cooperation' (NCCOP 1960: 38).

In 1960, the review of the NCCOP rest homes concluded that 'it would be a major tragedy if any of these . . . homes were to close down', and that 'serious thought should be given to the provision of more of them' (NCCOP 1960: 36,38). However, by the mid-1960s the 'experiment' was over. The NCCOP homes were transferred to hospitals, and there is no mention of the King Edward's Hospital Fund homes after the late 1950s in their annual reports. It appears that policy-makers were never again to give serious attention to the provision of rest homes.

Hospital discharge schemes

Over the last fifteen years, hospital discharge schemes have evolved, without any apparent awareness of their predecessors, as a community-based response to the problem of giving care and support to elderly people on discharge from hospital (Skeet 1970). Richards, writing in 1980, noted that 'the transition from the highly supportive environment of hospital to a home which may be extremely unsuitable for convalescence has been the subject of a number of research reports over the last decade' (Richards 1980: 1)

In brief, research studies, conducted primarily by the voluntary sector and community health councils (see, for example, Skeet 1970; Amos 1973; Continuing Care Project 1975; Singh *et al* 1979; Williamson 1985) found that many discharges from hospital were poorly planned, and that consequently elderly patients returned home from hospital with unmet needs. The studies concluded that, notwithstanding the emphasis in geriatric medicine on the social as well as the medical needs of its patients, the appointment of liaison nursing staff in some hospitals, the network of day hospitals, and the wide range of statutory and non-statutory domiciliary services available to elderly people, the provision of transitional care on discharge from hospital was still, in many areas of the country, more fortuitous than guaranteed.

During the 1970s, in response to these research findings, the voluntary sector became involved in the co-ordination of those involved in the discharge process and in the provision of post-discharge support (Richards 1980; Landsberger 1985). Slowly, a patchwork of hospital discharge schemes was established around the country. In 1985, three of the main voluntary organizations working in the field received short-term funding under the government's 'Helping the Community to Care' programme to co-ordinate eighteen demonstration 'home from hospital' projects (DHSS 1984, 1986a). These projects are described as focusing on the management of hospital discharge, the transition of elderly patients from hospital to their own homes, the provision of personal care and support by trained volunteers to patients and their families in the immediate post-discharge period, and the prevention of readmission to hospital. In South Glamorgan, a hospital discharge service is co-ordinated by the voluntary sector, with funding from the Second European Poverty Programme. The service employs paid 'settlement aides' to travel home from hospital with elderly patients and provide intensive support for the first few critical days after discharge. This is then followed by less formal, longer-term volunteer support. The service describes itself as attempting to prevent the necessity for readmissions due more to socio-economic than medical circumstances, aiming to complement the input of other support services, and to assist the elderly person to become independent in the community. The service also aims to facilitate collaboration between health and social and between hospital and community services.

Discussion

A crucial question, from a policy perspective, is why has one form of post-discharge provision for elderly people been replaced by another? Why did the concept of rest homes not survive, and, why have both forms of provision remained at the level of an 'experiment', and peripheral to mainstream service provision?

What happened to rest homes?

Dickson, writing about one ot the NCCOP homes (Springbok home), explains the demise of the experimental rest homes thus:

> the gap which Springbok had been designed to fill was closing of its own accord. In 1954, the Ministry of Health made it clear that local authorities were expected to cater for the infirm elderly, and thereby encouraged the development of domiciliary services and sheltered housing, with more ground floor provision within Part III accommodation. At the same time, great advances had been made in the field of geriatric medicine in general, and with rehabilitation in particular.
> (Dickson 1978)

Dickson's assumption appears to be that the blending of health care and social support necessary for the adequate care of 'partly sick and partly well' old people in their homes after discharge from hospital had somehow happened by virtue of the post-war developments of the NHS's hospitals and the local authority's social services. In fact, the self-evident separateness of these developments was one important stimulus for the adoption of 'community care' policies from the late 1950s. 'Community care' was meant to represent the integration of care in a non-hospital setting. However, whilst health and local authority domiciliary services *have* clearly developed in the period under discussion, the latest evidence from reports by the Audit Commission and the Cumberlege Committee suggests that, as a concept, community care has made little progress as a result of the institutional and professional apartheid that exists between health and social services in 'the community' as well as between hospitals and these services (Audit Commission 1986; DHSS 1986b).

The demise of the rest homes and the assumed disappearance of the need for which they evolved may to some extent be explained by the masking effect of two kinds of rather hopeful rhetoric — one about the integrative functions of 'development' and the other about the totality of provision through 'community care'. The strength of the appeal of such rhetoric is probably due both to considerations of cost and to the intractability of the institutional, budgetary, and professional divisions of the health and social services. Indeed, the review of NCCOP homes, quoted earlier, noted that from the very beginning 'the Ministry of Health were not eager for these experiments to be made fearing administrative difficulties and possibly a demand for increased accommodation at a time when finance was not available' (NCCOP 1960: 31). Rather than tackle structural problems within and between the two systems, policy-makers took refuge in hopeful ideas about the availability of care and its integration in the community.

Dickson's second assumption was that changing medical practice in rehabilitation techniques made the need for a half-way institutional arrangement for elderly people between hospital and home somehow obsolete. There is no gainsaying the fact that developments in geriatrics and new approaches to rehabilitation have, as Dickson suggests, had a significant impact on the kind and severity of needs involved in the elderly person's hospital after-care. They have also had a considerable effect on the nature of progressive patient care of the elderly people in hospital (see Andrews and Brocklehurst 1987). Nevertheless, these developments have not, by themselves, necessarily removed the need for some of the more convalescent functions provided by the rest home: assistance with resettlement after a hospital stay, a 'health' environment in which to recover fully, and time for the necessary social arrangements to be made for returning home.

However, during the 1950s the movement against convalescence was gathering momentum, and the demise of rest homes can also be seen as the organizational expression of the general decline of convalescence as a medical concept. It seems that, as a care category, elderly people have been swept along by a medical tide that was busy redefining the optimum regimen for medical recovery. Convalescence as a form of provision was no longer considered medically necessary for other age-groups: indeed, it became medically fashionable to advocate activity rather than bed rest, and rapid return to customary tasks rather than legitimized idleness. The elderly were included in this new vogue without further thought.

The question that needs to be raised is whether such developments have left the specific needs of frail elderly people unaddressed. There is first the growing number and proportion of very old frail individuals among those of pensionable age (Age Concern 1981), and the changing patterns of household formation and family support (Rossiter and Wicks 1982). There is also the relatively poorer housing and living conditions of the elderly population, compared with other age-groups (Wheeler 1986). The care implications of reduced lengths of stay in hospital also need to be considered, since elderly people take longer to recover from illness and from medical and surgical intervention than do young people. The trend to shorter periods of hospitalization has unequivocally been presented as an achievement, with rarely any accompanying discussion of the implications for patients during their hospital stay, or their post-discharge experience. The enquiry into convalescent treatment in 1959 had the foresight to point out that whilst the medical need for convalescence may have diminished, the 'need to free a hospital bed, to provide less costly in-patient care or to delay the discharge home for social reasons may not' (Ministry of Health 1959: 9). The demise of rest homes, along with the majority of convalsecent homes and NHS convalescent beds, meant that these needs would have to be addressed through alternative provision. It is in this context that the emergence of hospital discharge schemes must be viewed.

The rest home concept must also have been affected by the changes in thinking about institutional forms of provision which were occurring in this country from the end of the 1950s (Goffman 1961; Townsend 1962). The total institution, with all its drawbacks, represented a kind of integration between medical and social care. From the 1960s, it was being increasingly challenged. The ideology of 'community care' was gaining force, stimulated perhaps most importantly by considerations of cost, but also by ideas surrounding personal independence, family and community links, and the superiority in humane terms of a small-scale, domestic environment. In this sense, the transition from the institutional form of the rest home to the domiciliary emphasis of the hospital discharge scheme mirrored the general trend in social service provision which begun in the 1970s.

Why hospital discharge schemes?

Some ten or so years after the demise of the rest home experiment, hospital discharge schemes emerged to plug a 'yawning gap' (Potterton 1984) between hospital and community services, raising questions about whether gaps between service provision and need had reappeared, or whether, as hinted, they had never really disappeared, but had simply been socially deconstructed. Ostensibly, the gap plugged by hospital discharge schemes is different from that which was covered by the rest homes. The requisite care and support services do exist, but the problem is defined as one of liaison and timing. Schemes are commonly described as covering the communication gap that exists between hospital and community, a gap that results in delays in the establishing or re-establishing of statutory domiciliary services after a period of hospitalization. However, this description, and indeed hospital discharge schemes themselves, may mask other dimensions of the gap — namely, an inadequate level or range of statutory service provision. We look at both of these dimensions in turn.

Statutory resource levels

Richards (1980), in an Age Concern action guide on hospital after-care schemes, suggested that patients leaving hospital were falling through the net of the caring services partly because of the wide range of different people involved, working in many disciplines and employed by various bodies, but also because 'the community services are . . . overstretched and unable to provide adequate home support'. Age Concern Wales, in recommending the initiation of hospital discharge schemes in the principality, 'considered the urgent situation created by the curtailing of public expenditure and its effect on services for the elderly provided by Health and Social Services'. (Age Concern Wales 1979). It may be, then, that, in addition to communication and liaison problems, the time-lag between hospital and community services provision is due to the escalating needs of an increasingly elderly population. Official policy statements on the care of elderly people present their rising numbers as problematic, and suggest that the increasing 'burden' of the frail among them somehow inevitably means overstretched statutory resources and the need for the voluntary and informal sectors to step in (Phillipson and Walker 1986). Such a view can be challenged as resting upon a particular ideological perspective on ageing. To quote Jefferys (1987), 'it is only a failure to recognise that it is our sense of values and not an insoluble problem of limited means which prevents us from recognising that we already possess ample resources for the task in hand'. It is the social position given to elderly people that perhaps ultimately explains why solutions to the problem of their hospital discharge and after-care have usually taken the form of temporary measures tacked on to the statutory services from the voluntary sector, rather than specific services geared to their needs. No other explanation is adequate to account for their relative neglect compared with younger people with special needs. It contrasts, for example, with the statutory after-care arrangements for mothers and their newly born babies on return from hospital.

Range of statutory provision

From our preliminary research, it is clear that hospital discharge schemes are providing a form of care that is qualitatively different to that provided by the statutory health and social care services. To describe such schemes as simply filling a time gap left by the statutory services is to underestimate their innovative feature, which is to provide a form of support designed around individual needs rather than slotting individuals into existing services and existing categories whether medical or social. In the early days of the welfare state it was assumed that proper classification and accurate diagnosis would enable elderly people to be divided into those whose needs were medical, and therefore the responsibility of the health services, and those whose needs were social, and therefore the responsibility of the local authority. This assumption led to the development of administrative and professional structures which turned out to be ill-equipped to provide for the intertwined needs of frail elderly people. Both rest homes and hospital discharge schemes can be seen as imaginative forms of provision that evolved in response to the unclassifiable and ambiguous needs of those who are 'partly sick and partly well' on their discharge from hospital. It could, however, be argued that it was just this innovative feature of rest homes that hampered their development: the administrative and professional rigidities of health and social services could not adapt to a form of provision that required intersectorial collaboration and joint decision-making.

The emergence of hospital discharge schemes — and the growing number of private nursing homes for elderly people — hint at the need to re-examine yet another aspect of the revised medical orthodoxy that rationalized the demise of rest homes: the diminishing need for convalescence. Our preliminary research in South Glamorgan has suggested that hospital discharge schemes, in deploying 'settlement aides', are seeking to create a convalescing environment in the home for the elderly person returning from hospital. It may well be asked then to what extent the need for convalescence for elderly people has disappeared. Furthermore, does their experience imply that the appropriate place of convalescence has shifted from hospital to home? It would be useful to know, for example, to what extent the elderly who can afford to pay, 'buy in' a period of convalescence at a private home or, by employing others on a temporary basis, in their own homes (see Midwinter 1987). Our research suggests the need for a re-evaluation of past and present views and practice concerning convalescence.

Conclusion

From this brief description and historical comparison of rest homes and hospital discharge schemes, what can be learned about social policy development for elderly people on discharge from hospital? Over a period of thirty years, one model of care for elderly people discharged from hospital has replaced another. The transition from 'model one' (the rest home) to 'model two' (the hospital discharge scheme) followed the trends in other forms of social provision, in moving from an institutional to a domiciliary setting, from a high-cost to a low-cost solution that relies increasingly on low-paid workers and unpaid volunteers. Changing medical theories concerning convalescence have coincided with such transitions; so too have the ways in which needs have been defined, and in part deconstructed.

The main and pessimistic conclusion to be drawn is that the main statutory care system found no place for either model of discharge care. Both rest homes and hospital discharge schemes have been peripheral and impermanent forms of provision. Their voluntary status symbolizes the low level of policy attention that the issue of the discharge of older people has received. That status has enabled policy-makers to avoid the more fundamental task of tackling the institutional and professional blockages that impede a smooth transition from hospital to home and satisfactory convalescence for frail elderly people. Rest homes were described as 'experimental'; currently hospital discharge schemes are often depicted as demonstration projects. The question of what they are demonstrating is not answered, perhaps because it is not meant to be. What can be seen now with hospital discharge schemes is the fiction of a 'pilot project', a device that enables government to get away with short bursts of highly visible action, without tackling the more complex, underlying problems of the organization of care for vulnerable, marginal groups such as frail elderly people.

Is this too cynical and pessimistic a conclusion? With the current widespread disillusionment with community care policies and the Griffiths review of community care, is it possible to imagine a new integrated care system for frail elderly people evolving (Griffiths 1988)? Could those engaged in such a system genuinely learn the lessons offered first by the experimental rest homes and then by the pilot discharge schemes? Can the system defects which have given rise to the care gap be eliminated by integrating, as a permanent and securely funded resource, the innovative, tried, and tested schemes evolved by the voluntary sector?

Note

1. The authors would like to acknowledge the help and co-operation of Teresa Rees, joint evaluator of the South Glamorgan Hospital Discharge Service, Robert Taylor, Director of South Glamorgan Care for the Elderly, Julia O'Brien, and the other staff of the Hospital Discharge Service. The South Glamorgan Care for the Elderly Hospital Discharge Service and its

evaluation are funded by the European Community, the Welsh Office, South Glamorgan Health Authority, and South Glamorgan County Council. The project is one of ninety-one pilot projects in the Second European Programme to Combat Poverty. The evaluation of the Service is sub-contracted to the Social Research Unit, Department of Social Studies, University College, Cardiff.

References

Adams, G. (1954) 'Betwixt and between. A recovery home for the old', *Lancet* 2: 486–8.

Age Concern (1981) *Profiles of the Elderly: Their Use of the Social Services*, London Age Concern England.

Age Concern Wales (1979) 'Home from Hospital Project grant application submitted to Carnegie Trust', Cardiff: Age Concern Wales.

Amos, G. (1973) *Care is Rare*, London: Age Concern.

Andrews, K. and Brocklehurst, J. (1987) *British Geriatric Medicine in the 1980s*, London: King Edward's Hospital Fund for London.

Audit Commission (1986) *Making a Reality of Community Care*, London: HMSO.

Bosanquet, N. (1978) *A Future for Old Age*, London: Temple Smith/New Society.

Continuing Care Project (1975) *Going home?*, Birmingham: Continuing Care Project.

DHSS (1984) 'Helping the community to care', Press Release 84/218, London: DHSS Information Division.

DHSS (1986a) *Annual Report of the NHS for England*, London: HMSO.

DHSS (1986b) *Neighbourhood nursing — a focus for care*, London: HMSO.

Dickson, N. (1978) 'An alternative to the service "too young to benefit from lessons in its own history"', *Health and Social Services Journal*, 3 November: 1254–5.

Drain, G. (1957) 'Convalescence and the Hospital Service', *The Hospital*, May: 315–20.

Goffman, E. (1961) *Asylums: Essays on the Social Situation of Mental Patients and Other Inmates*, New York: Anchor Books, Doubleday & Co.

Griffiths, R. (1988) *Community Care: Agenda for Action*, A Report to the Secretary of State for Social Services, London: HMSO.

Jefferys, M. (1987) 'An ageing Britain — What is its future?', *Geriatric Nursing and Home Care* July: 19–24.

King Edward's Hospital Fund (1954) *Recovery Homes*, London: King Edward's Hospital Fund.

Landsberger, B. (1985) *Long term care for the elderly*, London: Croom Helm.

Means, R. and Smith, R. (1985) *The development of Welfare Services for Elderly People*, London: Croom Helm.

Midwinter, E. (1987) *Caring for Cash: The Issue of Private Domiciliary Care*, London: Centre for Policy on Ageing.

Ministry of Health (1959) *Convalescent Treatment: Report of a Working Party*, SO Code No. 32–463, London: HMSO.

National Corporation for the Care of Old People (NCCOP) (1960), *Appendi to Thirteenth Annual Report for the Year Ended 30th September 1960*, London: NCCOP.

National Corporation for the Care of Old People (1961) *Fourteenth Annual Report for the Year ended 30th September, 1961*, London: NCCOP.

Phillipson, C. and Walker, A. (1986) *Ageing and Social Policy*, Aldershot: Gower.

Potterton, D. (1984) 'The Yawning Gap', *Nursing Times* 8 August: 34–5.

Richards, T. (1980) *Hospital after-care schemes*, London: Age Concern, England.

Rossiter, C. and Wicks, M. (1982) *Crisis or Challenge: Family Care, Elderly People and Social Policy*, London: Study Commission on the Family.

Russell, J. (1986) 'Hospital discharge schemes for the elderly: policy, practice and evaluation', Report of a one day research seminar held on 21 November at University College, Cardiff.

Singh, J., Hogg, G., and Hogg, C. (1979) *Leaving Hospital: A report on the Experience of Elderly People Leaving Hospital* London: Victoria Community Health Council.

Skeet, M. (1970) *Home from Hospital*, London: Macmillan.

Townsend, P. (1962) *The Last Refuge: A Survey of Residential Institutions and Homes for the Aged in England and Wales*, London: Routledge & Kegan Paul.

Townsend, P. (1981) 'The Structured Dependency of the Elderly: the Creation of Social Policy in the 20th Century', *Ageing and Society* 1 (1): 5–28.

Wheeler, R. (1986) 'Housing policy and elderly people', in C. Phillipson and A. Walker eds *Ageing and Social Policy*, Aldershot: Gower.

Williamson, V. (1985) *Who really cares: A Survey on the Aftercare of Elderly Patients Discharged from Acute Hospital*, Hove: Brighton Community Health Council.

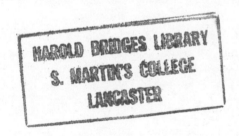

Chapter thirteen

Black Old Women, Disability, and Health Carers[1]

Elaine Cameron, Helen Evers, Frances Badger and Karl Atkin

Introduction

This chapter focuses on black old women who are disabled and black women who are carers of older disabled family members. It explores some of the emergent issues and themes from a broader research project currently in progress in Central Birmingham Health Authority (Evers *et al* forthcoming). This project is looking at community services to, and needs of, physically disabled, frail elderly, and elderly mentally infirm people living at home. It incorporates an exploratory sociological study of how black disabled elders perceive health and illness, how disability is construed and responded to in the context of their social networks, and the nature of contacts with statutory and other helping agencies.

For the present purposes and following current convention, 'black' refers to people who are of Afro-Caribbean or Asian descent.

Why focus on black disabled old women and their health carers?

The reasons are, of course, many and varied, touching on issues both of academic and practical concern.

First, there is a growing body of literature on black people and health and on black elders (Bhalla and Blakemore 1981; Barker 1984; Norman 1985; Holland and Lewando-Hundt 1987). However, although some attention has been drawn specifically to black people who are disabled (RADAR 1984; GLAD 1987), this remains a neglected area, as does the situation of black old women. Moreover, with few exceptions (for example, Donovan 1986), there has been little systematic research exploring black women's and men's perspectives, and this is mirrored by the relatively slow development of conceptual frameworks to address these areas within gerontology, sociology, and women's studies.

Second, gender, along with race, age, and class, is a major variable in social stratification. British gerontology has begun to analyse the significance of sex and gender in old age (Peace 1986), but to date has paid less attention to ethnic minorities.

Third, there is mounting evidence that ethnic minority groups are disadvantaged in terms of health in all age-groups (Townsend and David-son 1982; Whitehead 1987). Furthermore, black people are more likely to have disabling conditions earlier in old age than white people and to undergo 'premature ageing' (Bhalla and Blakemore, 1981). As the prevalence of disability in older women is higher than in older men (Harris *et al* 1971, Hunt, 1978), old black women are likely to be a group with relatively high rates of disability.

Fourth, demographic trends indicate an imminent steep growth in the numbers of older people of Afro-Caribbean and Asian descent. At the moment, the proportion of black elders of pensionable age is small, but the group aged between 45 and pensionable age is much larger, as Table 13.1 shows.

Table 13.1 Age and place of birth, women and men in age-group as a percentage of total UK women and men in age-group

| | New Commonwealth and Pakistan (excluding Caribbean) | | Caribbean | |
	F	M	F	M
45–pensionable age	1.80	2.26	0.90	1.00
Pensionable age and over	0.72	0.80	0.16	0.17

Source: 1981 Census of England and Wales, HMSO.

Fifth, surveys, including our own, have shown that black women and men are underrepresented among those receiving community health and social services (Bhalla and Blakemore 1981; Donaldson 1986; Holland and Lewando-Hundt 1987; McFarland *et al.* 1987).[2] Inaccessibility of services to black people makes for the 'triple jeopardy' situation that Norman (1985) so vividly describes. If black old people are more likely to be disabled yet less likely to be receiving care from the statutory services, then who are their carers? Is it likely that, as with the majority white-community, carers are more often the women?

British health and welfare policy has tended to ignore the special needs of ethnic minority groups. The adoption of a 'colour blind' stance in policy and practice has meant that services provided have been, in effect, discriminatory. Furthermore, in the current political and economic climate, all old people, and particularly black disabled old women, are likely to be among the most vulnerable.

Research which addresses the above issues may provide data which help services make informed decisions about how best to serve the community. This research is important now, not just because of the current shift in emphasis to community care, but also because of the imminent increase in numbers and potential 'needs' of black elders. Further, as most of the black communities are spatially concentrated, there will be an increased localized impact of demographic changes and needs, with important implications for services already overstretched in the inner city. This chapter draws from research which has begun to address some of these issues.

The Community Care Research Project

Service providers from district nursing, health visiting for the elderly, community psychiatric nursing for the elderly, social work, occupational therapy, and home-help teams were interviewed, using a structured schedule, about their knowledge of, and their work with, a random sample of clients and patients currently on their case-loads. A smaller sample of these clients was subsequently visited and interviewed in depth about many aspects of their lives, including thier contacts with services.

Disabled adults of Afro-Caribbean and of Asian descent were shown to be underrepresented among the clients and patients, but with social services having higher proportions than health services. The average proportion of black clients across community services' teams (excluding the home-help service) was approximately 7 per cent and seemed much too low given the population structure of central Birmingham, where around 20 per cent of the total population of 180,000 live in households where the head is of New Commonwealth or Pakistani origin.

Having found black people of both sexes to be underrepresented in the survey of community services, we decided to study the views of older Asians and Afro-Caribbeans on health, illness, disability, and service provision in greater detail, by interviewing a population-based sample of physically disabled people who may or may not be known to services. We also wanted to explore the parallels and differences between black and white elders in terms of perceptions of health and illness and their support networks.

Defining disability

Defining and measuring disability, despite widespread attention and research, is still a problematic area. The major contributions which have been made (for example, Townsend 1967, Jefferys *et al.* 1969, Harris *et al.* 1971, Agerholm 1975, Blaxter 1976, Bury and Wood 1978,

WHO 1980, Duckworth 1983, Locker 1983), have provided various helpful conceptual frameworks as well as highlighting major practical difficulties of operationalizing such concepts. Most useful for these purposes is the widely drawn distinction between impairment, disability, and handicap and the nature of their interrelationship. Basically, 'impairment' refers to loss or abnormality of physical or psychological function, 'disability' to the resulting lack of ability to perform 'normal' activities, and 'handicap' to the disadvantage which stems from impairment or disability.

The definitions in the study which were used to select the client group relate to 'disability' and were chosen so as to identify, in a fairly simple way, groups of people who have mobility problems which affect their everyday lives (Figure 13.1). Those with primarily sensory impairments were excluded from the study.

Physically disabled and frail elderly people, for the purposes of the survey, are those who have any of the following characteristics:

1. are bedfast;
2. have significant difficulty in walking or going up and down stairs;
3. use walking aids or wheelchairs;
4. have chronic sickness, any other illness or some permanent disability which STOPS or SIGNIFICANTLY LIMITS their working, or getting about, or taking care of themselves.

To be 'eligible' for our study, the individual will have had one or more of the above characteristics for at least SIX MONTHS FROM NOW.

Figure 13.1 Definitions of patients/clients included in the survey

In the area of handicap, contextual factors and 'meanings' become especially important; it is the sphere in which a physical condition takes on social significance. It is the sphere, Locker suggests, in which various resources — physical, cognitive, material, and social — may be brought to bear by the individual. Locker argues that it is at present only possible to work with indicators of handicap, such as income, social isolation, and so on, that no adequate measuring instrument has yet been developed; and moreover, that these indicators address important aspects, but not 'handicap' in its entirety (Locker 1983).

Research methods

We focused on Asians because they form the largest ethnic minority group in this part of Birmingham (Sparkhill and Sparkbrook areas), and because other evidence indicated that this group was least likely to know about existing services (Holland and Lewando-Hundt, 1987). A practical but important consideration was the ability to identify Asians by name from our sampling frame, records from five general practices in Central Birmingham Health Authority one of which was used as a pilot.[3]

Samples were selected randomly from each of four groups: Asian men and Asian women aged 55 years and over; non-Asian men and non-Asian women aged 65 years and over (see Table 13.2). It was hoped that the non-Asian groups would yield some disabled Afro-Caribbeans. The difference in lower age-limits would afford inter-ethnic group 'comparability' in terms of health states following findings from an earlier study (Blakemore 1983). Comparison is crucial to gauge which factors can be attributed to the contingencies of ethnicity. Letters were sent to those in the sample (n = 337) on practice-headed notepaper and written in Gujarati, Hindi, Punjabi, Urdu, and English. In the absence of a negative response to the letter, this was followed two to three weeks later by a visit and screening interview to establish if the respondent was disabled according to the broad definitions we were using. If so, the interviewer continued with the main interview schedule.

Table 13.2 Overall Response Rates

	Asian		Non-Asian		Totals		Total
	F	M	F	M	F	M	
Interviews	38	46	41	37	79	83	162
Non response[a] (all causes)	55	54	27	39	82	93	175
Totals	93	100	68	76	161	176	337
Response rates (%)	40.9	46.0	60.3	48.7	49.1	47.2	48.1

Note: a. Reasons for non-response were died, gone away, address not found, not known at address, refusal, and non-contact after three calls.

Table 13.3 Total Numbers Interviewed

	Asian		Afro-Caribbean		Non-Asian/non Afro-Caribbean		Totals		Total
	F	M	F	M	F	M	F	M	
Disabled	14	19	2	7	20	13	36	39	
Not disabled	24	27	3	0	16	17	43	44	
Total	38	46	5	7	36	30	79	83	162

Interviews with those who were disabled continued, where possible, with more broad-ranging discussions. These focused on perceptions of health states, meanings of disability, biographies, experiences and expectations of old age, features of everyday life, patterns of family and service care, and the nature of any service contacts and referral pathways.

Table 13.4 Age and sex of disabled elders

	Asian		Afro-Caribbean		Non-Asian/non Afro-Caribbean		Totals		Total
Age (years)	F	M	F	M	F	M	F	M	
ɔ4 years and under	1	0	0	0	0	0	1	0	1
55–64	4	12	0	1	0	1	4	14	18
65–74	6	5	1	6	8	1	15	12	27
75–84	2	2	1	0	9	10	12	12	24
85–94	1	0	0	0	3	1	4	1	5
	14	19	2	7	20	13	36	39	75

In a few selected cases, further interviews were held with the respondent, other family members, and carers. Interviews were tape-recorded where respondents gave permission, which they did in most cases.

The overall response rates and the numbers of Asian and non-Asian elders in the study are given in Tables 13.2, 13.3, and 13.4.

Research challenges

Prior to outlining some of the themes which are emerging, it is interesting to consider some of the particular challenges we encountered and how we addressed them.

Members of the research team were white; thus every effort was needed to draw on the expertise of black community care workers and researchers. Asian interviewers and interpreters were used and their own experiences and perceptions similarly drawn on. The individual-centred interview, which also reflects the typical services response, is likely to be an inappropriate and alien research mode here; as far as possible open-ended discussions and interviews in family settings were used.

Research which focuses on black people is in danger of reinforcing implicit or explicit racism or of being patronizing. Social researchers are faced with the difficult problem of the management of their power position. We have found no easy solution to these weighty issues. The lower refusal rate, as distinct from other reasons for non-response, for the Asian and Afro-Caribbean groups compared to the non Asian/non Afro-Caribbean group perhaps reflects this power relationship.

Another challenge concerns 'meaning', a central issue for social science by virtue of its key role in social relations, and important here in connection with exploring the concept of 'handicap'. In our project the key role of the interviewer as a 'filter' in attempting to ascertain meaning, for example of handicap, is made more difficult by the possibility or likelihood that the experiences and frames of reference of the researcher and black respondents are different in major and fundamental respects. This necessitates a testing of sociological insight, and at the outset sets important limitations.

The Findings: some themes and some figures

The findings from the study are to be reported in full elsewhere (Evers *et al* forthcoming). The focus here is on four selected themes: stereotypes, the position of the aged in society, expectations of old age, and the 'misfit' between clients and services. Following this will be a consideration of the perspectives of black women on caring and being cared for, their perspectives on disability, and the services' response to them.

Stereotypes

Our research, like other studies, shows some support for the common stereotypes of the situation of black elders. Thus, for example, black people usually lived in self-supporting extended families and seemed less likely to need services' support. However, these notions are clearly oversimple and therefore misleading. There were older black people who lived alone or whose relatives lived at a distance, and some were childless. Living with families did not necessarily mean that service support was not needed. Table 13.5 gives the household composition for the different ethnic groups. It can be seen that non-Asians were far more likely to be living alone or just with a spouse than were Asians.

Table 13.5 Household composition of all respondents

	Asian			Afro-Caribbean			Non-Asian/non-Afro-Caribbean		
	F	M	Total	F	M	Total	F	M	Total
Lives alone	1	2	3	1	2	3	20	9	29
Lives with spouse only	3	4	7	2	2	4	4	11	15
Lives with other(s)	34	40	74	2	3	5	12	10	22
Total	38	46	84	5	7	12	36	30	66

There was enormous diversity both in life histories and current circumstances within and between Afro-Caribbean and Asian groups, and this partly reflects patterns of migration and settlement. There were those who came to seek work, usually men among the Asian community and both women and men among the Afro-Caribbean; others came to join families or to settle as exiles or refugees. Some had spent many years in this country while others came when already old (Barker 1984). Furthermore, changing life-styles from one generation to the next also affected family structures: children moved away for education or jobs, or set up their own families.

Mrs Bi, a woman interviewed in our study, illustrated a break with the popular stereotype of household and lifestyle. A Muslim, aged 69, she came from Kenya to join her daughter nineteen years ago. Among her other health problems she suffered from severe arthritis, and her disability restricted her to living downstairs. Her daughter, with whom she lived, was her main carer. Mrs. Bi and her daughter were quite isolated. Both women occupied marginal roles because of a complex interplay of factors, including physical disability, and social and cultural pressures. Contrary to the stereotype, moreover, Mrs Bi had some contact with services and her daughter had requested day care for her, and adaptations to the house.

The position of old people in society

All old people, black and white, occupy a relatively low position in the social structure and the associated patterns of disadvantage have been well documented and variously explained (Norman 1980; Walker 1980; Townsend 1981; Phillipson 1982; Fennell *et al*, 1988). Some disadvantages, such as bad housing and environment, poverty and low income, and social isolation are more amenable to identification and measurement than others such as low social status, relative lack of power, and control of relatively few resources. All such diasdvantages, however, may be further exacerbated by increased susceptibility to poor health.

Black old people, however, tend to be even further disadvantaged: for example, for a variety of reasons their incomes are likely to be lower in old age than those of white elderly people (Norman 1985). The women in particular have least access to and control over financial resources (Cook and Watt 1987), especially in later life. Black old people are perhaps more likely to spend their old age in deprived inner-city environments.

Isolation is another aspect of old age that particularly affects black older people. They are likely to be more isolated by limited mobility and language barriers: in our study, none of the thirty-eight Asian women and only fifteen of the forty-six Asian men were fluent in English. In addition, many have experienced major disruptions which leave them feeling marooned, sometimes with no close kin nearby or away from friends and familiar surroundings.

Mr Khan, a 63 year-old man who came from Pakistan in the 1950s, had no close family and lived alone in a warden-controlled flat. This is how he described his feelings of isolation: 'I got no-one . . . no. . . my district is nowhere, I got nobody.'

Perhaps the key feature, which is central to the structural disadvantages that old black people face, is the one that affects all black people — racism. Racism, in all its various forms and expressions, affects the lives of black people, often in ways of which they are not fully conscious. In this study very few black people spoke about it as a continuing experience. When the subject arose it was usually mentioned in the context of somewhat detached past experiences such as immigration, employment, or housing. For example, one elderly Jamaican-born man said: 'No-one wants old black people coming to live near them, you've got to be realistic these days.'

That experiences of racism were seldom discussed by our respondents may be due in part to the fact that the interviewer was sometimes white, or that it was painful to recall racist experiences. It is also possible that disabled older black people, because they were less visible in public places, face fewer potentially racist situations. Certainly, it was not uncommon for old black people to talk about avoiding stressful situations. It is ironic that disabled elders, who may be one of the black groups most disadvantaged by structural racism, may also be least able or willing to speak of it.

Expectations of old age

In the study, black and white elders shared gloomy stereotypes of old age as a time of restricted outlook and activity, poorer health and mobility, and increased dependency.

Spending old age in Britain had additional problems for many black people. Some came expecting to return 'home' (see Anwar 1979), and, though they still wanted to, felt trapped here. Some could not go back because they did not have enough money for the fare, or because their children, who have settled here, would not be able to afford to visit them. For others it was because the place they left had changed or there was no-one left there to return to. For still others, going back would mean loss of face.

Mr Campbell, a 71 year-old Jamaican born man disabled by diabetes said: 'I came with two legs, I can't go back with one.'

Black elders, most of whom have experienced major disruptions during their lives, also faced old-age experiences different from those they had traditionally grown up with. Some felt they had not 'earned' their dependency in the established cultural way, because they had been separated from those children during the years when they would normally have provided social and economic support for them. Others faced situations where the children had moved away or could offer limited support only.

'Misfit' between clients and services

Another finding was that the 'fit' between all old people's needs and community care services was often imperfect, haphazard, and inflexible. Referral networks into and between services did not easily allow for effective service support. Clearly a system which works ineffectively to meet the needs of its majority white clients is even less likely to begin to address, in a sensitive way, the area of black people's needs, even if this largely 'invisible' need were to be presented to it.

Black women as carers

Just as in the white community, women proved to be the mainstay of the informal care provided to black elders who were frail or disabled, as Table 13.6 shows.

Table 13.6 Main lay carers of disabled elders

Carer	Cared for						
	Asian		Afro-Caribbean		Total female carers	Non-Asian/non Afro-Caribbean		Total female carers
	F	M	F	M		F	M	
n =	14	19	2	7		20	13	
Wife	—	11	—	4		—	4	
Daughter	1	1	0	1		8	1	
Daughter-in-law	4	2	0	0		0	0	
Other female relative	2	0	0	0		0	3	
Female non-relative	0	0	0	0	26	3	1	20
					Total male carers			*Total male carers*
Husband	4	—	2	—		0	—	
Son	1	2	0	0		2	0	
Other male relative	0	0	0	0		2	0	
Male non-relative	0	0	0	0	9	1	0	5
No helper	1	1	0	1		1	2	
Missing information	1	2	0	1		3	2	

Perhaps the most striking feature of the study was the enormous resilience, versatility, resourcefulness, and social and individual strengths that both black and white women carers displayed, very often in extremely difficult circumstances, and lacking additional support. The case of Mrs Thomas is one of many which illustrates this point.

Mrs Thomas was 52 and was the main carer of her 66 year-old husband, who came to Britain in 1961 from Anguilla. Mr Thomas was well until three years earlier when a stroke left him unable to walk or care for himself. After his discharge from hospital Mrs Thomas looked after him, unsupported, for two years.

The many disadvantages, penalties, and limitations associated with a female caring-role found ready examples in this study. What was noticeable was the centrality of this role in the day-to-day lives of carers, and the 'pushes' and 'pulls' which interact in the complex balance between *wanting* to care, because of emotional bonds, and *having* to care through lack of perceived or actual alternative support.

In our study, Mrs Bond was the daughter and main carer of Mrs Bryant, an 81 year-old white widow who suffered from arthritis and had recently become incontinent. Following Mrs Bryant's recent fall, both women moved to a ground floor flat so that the daughter could care for her. Mrs Bond was divorced, had no children, and worked full time, though nearing retirement. When she was interviewed, Mrs Bryant was receiving no services and was feeling very isolated. Mrs Bond found caring for her mother very exhausting but was clearly devoted to her.

Black women carers, however, often faced particular difficulties over and above those faced by white women. Some were recent arrivals, facing culture shock and with little or no knowledge of the system or of how or where to seek support for the disabled person for whom they were caring. The case of Mrs Patel, who was 57 and came with her family to England in 1980 from Kenya via India, is an example. She had difficulties with mobility and self-care following an accident a year earlier in which she was knocked down by a car on a zebra crossing. She was brought home and taken to hospital by her son who had very little English, no-one in the family being aware of the ambulance emergency service. Her daughter-in-law, who was her main carer, could not speak English, and nobody in the immediate family knew about or had been told of any of the community services.

Many older women spoke more than one language, but not English. Many, for various reasons, had had little or no formal education, and the ability to read or write may not have the same significance in their countries of origin as it did in this country. Interpreter services were not as commonly available as many would have liked and both service providers and clients expressed dissatisfaction with those which did exist. Afro-Caribbeans too faced communication barriers.

Another disadvantage that black women faced in their role as carers was physical isolation: some were restricted to their houses through fear of an 'alien' outside world where their own norms, values, and social skills were often regarded as inappropriate, their behaviours in danger of mis-representation, or where they were confronted by many subtle expressions of racism. Bad weather and cultural taboos also contributed to the isolation of black women. These reduced the possibility of chance encounters: old black women were 'invisible' as were the disabled people they cared for.

The black women, moreover, were sometimes isolated or marginalized within their own cultural groups. Religious and voluntary groups, particu-larly Asian, tended to be male dominated, and not to accommodate 'deviant' individuals (for example, the divorced). For Asian women the new experience of caring for a disabled person, which typifies the 'individualized' response to disability in western society, was often an alien and unanticipated one.

Other stresses for older black women as carers also stemmed from changes in traditional family structures and role relationships. Women in their middle years caring for disabled parents or parents-in-law were also mothers of daughters who usually had been born in Britain and had often moved away from traditional ways via education, work, and sometimes marriage partners. This generation of black carers was often involved in role conflict. In the course of their day to day lives they could face a range of ambiguities in mediating between the different 'worlds' of the generation above and below theirs.

Another disadvantage was that older black women were likely to have limited access to financial resources. Many arrived with their families in Britain with little or no money, and shared with their menfolk the consequences of low-paid work, carrying minimal pension-rights. Whilst it was common for Asian families to pool their resources and help each other financially, women were often excluded from decision-making in these matters and also from the day-to-day handling of household finances. Black women carers, therefore, tended not to have the flexibility which some control over money matters could provide.

A final consideration was that where traditional care patterns existed, it was usually 'costly' to the daughter or daughter-in-law in a variety of ways. It could be in terms of education, of career prospects, of income, or of life chances and choices more generally.

A 66 year-old Asian widow, Mrs Sharma, who came from Africa in the 1960s, was severely disabled after a stroke in 1985. She lived with her son, daughter-in-law (who was her main carer), and two granddaughters. She was very dependent, day and night, needed help with toileting and feeding, and had difficulty speaking. Her daughter-in-law never left her except when she had relief care every two months. Despite help from services, her own life was severely restricted by her mother-in-law's ill health.

Our study showed that these 'costs' often began very early in life. Girls from Asian families were on occasions the ones who were needed to act as interpreters for their disabled grandparent.

Before moving on from 'carers', and also to avoid the pitfall of contributing to yet another stereotype, it is important to focus briefly on the minority of situations in which the main lay carer of a black disabled person was male (i.e. nine of the thirty-five cases known to have carers in this study). In some ways men, by stepping into a 'hands on' carer's role, which extended beyond the traditional support role relationship with an older family member, are vulnerable to even more pressures than women. Sociologically, these situations typify the effects of changing traditional family structures and the enduring capacity of individuals to adapt and cope in difficult times.

Mrs Desai was a pale thin women in her late sixties, confined to her bed because of a skeletal disorder. Her son had cared for her and his disabled father, who had died the previous year, for four years. His wife and daughters helped mainly with housework and preparing meals; but, because he was able to lift her, he always helped with toileting and bathing. The son said, 'Somebody told me if you look after your mother and father properly, God will look after you and your kids . . . This is my pilgrimage, you know'. (translation)

Black women cared for

When needing care because of their own disabilities, black old women and men look to their daughters or daughters-in-law, but many are childless or have no kin living nearby.

Mrs. Ali, for example, in her late sixties, lived with her husband in a modern ground-floor flat. A professional couple, they had no children nor other relatives in Britain. She was severely disabled with arthritis and had sciatica, eye problems, and anaemia. For many reasons they were relatively isolated: they belonged to just a small minority Christian Indian group in Birmingham and had infrequent contact with this community. Although she had a home help, district nurse contact, and aids to mobility, she felt very vulnerable with no family to care for her.

Even though many black elders who were disabled lived with their extended family, they could still be isolated or neglected within the home. The rest of the family could be out at work, for example, and the old person out of the sight of the rest of the community — and, of course, of the services.

The case of Mrs Desai, described earlier, was one example of the minority of cases (approximately one in four) where the bulk of day-to-day care fell on a man. More commonly men had a limited caring role, related to their language skills. A son or son-in-law was sometimes the one to accompany a disabled woman on visits to the GP, hospital or other help agency, and this could be inhibiting for the woman who could be reluctant fully to express personal details through a male relative.

Black people's perspectives on disability

This research has only begun to explore the central concern of meaning and its ascription to disabled states. The problem for researchers, that individuals cannot always talk about the 'meanings' of things in their lives, has already been noted, but what they do say is a useful starting-point. It is not easy adequately to disentangle meaning of disability from the complex that makes up each individual's situation. Nor is it easy to extrapolate those issues which relate to being 'black' from those which may be shared by all those with disabilities.

Some of the things that black disabled people and black carers spoke about — their 'public' and also their 'private' accounts (Cornwell 1984) were as follows. Some talked of stigmatizing aspects of disability which lead to isolation, restricted activities, and social life. This was often what they expected to happen to themselves and to be expected by their community. Others mentioned practical problems such as the inability to plait hair in the 'proper' way, put on or wear traditional dress, which was upsetting to some women and associated with a sense of loss of worth and embarrassment. Being disabled also could mean not visiting the mosque because of the inability to sit cross-legged in the customary way. It also meant not being able to return to visit family members in Pakistan.

Perhaps the most striking aspect of the responses of black women to disability, in their roles as carers, was its great variation. Although there were many common experiences, individual responses reflected particular configurations of factors affecting the caring situation. For example, in some cases the carer and old disabled person being cared for occupied similar social worlds, and shared similar values, beliefs, and role expectations. In such families there were likely to be common understandings about disability and the expected behaviour of those with it. This was not always related to age or generation; it was associated with individual life experiences and family structures.

In other cases, there was less common ground, either generally or in key areas to do with disability and caring relationships. Mrs Shah was a widow living in temporary accommodation while her son had been having alterations done to his house so that his mother could live with them. Mrs Shah's granddaughter was doing A levels at college but came to sleep with her grandmother most nights of the week. Mrs Shah said her granddaughter was not keen to do this.

Mrs Shah's daughter came in on alternate days to cook for her, but had had a different set of experiences through her work and her children and she had different expectations about her own old age and dependency. She was 50 years old and her own children had mostly grown up and moved away and she missed them. She told us, 'they [children] are more important to you than parents. . . . Getting older doesn't bother me at all, its leaving my family, the family going. You are busy with six children and now I've only me and one son at home.' Of the future she said, 'I say I won't be a burden on anybody. I'll go and live in a home when I'm old, when I reach old age.' Women from three generations in this family, then, each with a quite different set of life experiences, had few common perspectives on disability, dependency, and role relationships.

Given this variety, it is useful to consider disability and black perspectives at two analytical levels, which, though the distinction is artificial, may provide insights into the relationship between disability and handicap. At the level of the individual, but still within a specific wider socio-cultural context, account must be taken of each person's unique experiences through life and the particular configuration of characteristics that make up his or her current situation. This can provide greater understanding of what disability means to that individual, and help to identify and map the particular package of resources that he or she may bring to bear. At the structural level, certain broad patterns emerge. 'Blackness' emerges as a significant specific factor as the shared experiences, qualities, and disadvantages become apparent. At this level, the distribution of various resources between and within groups that are available to mitigate the handicap or disadvantage of disability can be identified — resources which are linked not only to cultural norms and values but also to structural divisions in society.

How did services respond to the needs of black women carers and old disabled black women?

Essentially the answer to this question was that they seemed to do very little. Community-care services were in touch with relatively few clients in these categories, and where there was contact the effectiveness of the response was often limited. Why was this so?

Very few of the community-care-service personnel were themselves black, and those few were usually in the lower ranks. Thus, they had little say in policy-making and little power or credibility outside their own sphere of work. It is ironic that the National Health Service, which continues to rely so heavily on low-paid black female labour, fails even to recognize or serve the needs of disabled black women.

Many service providers saw black clients as 'problem'- or awkward clients. Some brief quotations from survey interviews illustrate such common stereotypes.

District Nurse: 'We have problems with their customs — we have battles with diabetics during Ramadan.'

Social Worker: 'Afro-Caribbeans tend to enjoy ill health.

District Nurse: 'Blacks have a lower pain threshold.'

District Nurse: (about an elderly Asian man) 'They expect you to do it all; you have to bully them. They're very stubborn.'

Other comments, though gleaned unsystematically, were a reasonable representation of views held by community health and social services staff. Black clients, we were told, tended to make inappropriate or excessive requests, to be ignorant about the permanence of certain health problems, to be difficult to motivate, to not comply with treatment plans, to turn up late for appointments, to complicate things by having more than one date of birth or no marriage certificate — sadly, the list seemed endless.

The inappropriateness of the response of the services to the needs of old or disabled black people was seen, however, in the provision of unacceptable aids, adaptations, often costly, that were not used because they did not meet cultural requirements, and bath nurses turned away, because their help with washing was interpreted as unhygienic (rinsing not being done in the customary way) or as an invasion of personal privacy.

Of course, there were those working in community-care service teams — a minority it seemed, and more often social workers — who were aware of the particular disadvantages black people laboured under and of the shortcomings of the service they provided. Some social workers, particularly those in the team for physical handicap, showed awareness of the different meanings of disability within different cultures, and of the behaviours expected of black disabled adults and their carers. Such insights were often gained 'on the job' and sometimes through the experiences of black friends: against the odds, they did their best to deliver a sensitive service, often without management support. They acknowledged the failure of the services to offer the care that was required and the need for fundamental changes.

Nevertheless, how best to improve services is generally unclear. Extending communication about the service on offer is essential but not the whole answer. The extensive take-up of service initiatives such as specialized sheltered housing, Asian meals-on-wheels and Asian home-helps, shows that the need is there (Norman 1985). We need, however, to know much more about the quality of interaction between clients and services.

A fully effective service response to the needs of the black community would necessitate a fundamental shift in the wider political, ideological, economic, and social structure. In the mean time, the services can have less ambitious goals where smaller issues can be addressed. These include greater awareness on the part of service workers of local minority cultures, and, in this case particularly, the black people's perspectives on disability that may not coincide with those of the white majority or service providers.

Some conclusions, implications, and further directions for research

Black old women share many of the disadvantages that affect old white women, but they are further disadvantaged because of the colour of their skin. As carers or cared for, they are largely invisible to the wider society. Whilst the issue of education and race has been addressed by, among others, social scientists, educationalists, and politicians, the health of black people in later life had no comparable platform and remains off the agenda. Even recent emphasis on 'the problems of the inner city' focuses on youth and what is seen as an area of potential threat. Black old women do not have the dubious advantage of such a weighty stereotype.

The result is a service provision which is basically ethnocentric and discriminatory because it is geared to the white majority and makes little or no provision for minorities. The services are largely inaccessible to black elderly people, and furthermore tend to support and perpetuate stereotypes.

Black old women are also often disadvantaged within their own culture, and those who are disabled are particularly vulnerable. So too are those who are the mainstay of informal care if they are deviant in some way — for example, if they are divorced or without kin.

Demographic projections indicate an increase in the proportion of black elders, particularly women, in the elderly population over the next decade. Those who are disabled will be a growing client group. They will also mean more caring work for families, particularly female members. Research which provides greater understanding of black people's perceptions of impairment, disability, and handicap, and the meaning they attach to them, is important if services are to make informed planning initiatives for effective community care. In a small way this exploratory research has begun to address these issues.

Notes

1. This chapter is based on research commissioned by Central Birmingham Health Authority and funded by the Inner City Partnership Programme. It is a shortened version of a longer paper, the full version of which can be obtained from the authors on request. Acknowledgements to Inner City Partnership Programme for funding, Dr R.K. Griffiths, Director of Health Care Policy,

Central Birmingham Health Authority, and the subjects and service providers we interviewed.

2. Exceptions are use of general practitioner and some hospital services. Johnson *et al.* (1983) and Ebrahim *et al.* (1987) have shown that old people from ethnic minority groups are not under-users of these services. General practitioners and accident and emergency facilities are also perhaps the most easily accessible of health services.

3. We omitted those who might be considered 'elderly mentally infirm', for a range of reasons, though it is hoped to extend the research programme to focus on this key neglected group at a later date.

References

Agerholm, N. (1975) 'Handicaps and the handicapped: a nomenclature and classification of intrinsic handicaps', *Journal of the Royal Society of Health* 95: 3–8.

Anwar, M. (1979) *The Myth of Return, Pakistanis in Britain*, London: Heinemann.

Barker, J. (1984) *Black and Asian Old People in Britain* (Research perspectives on Ageing), Mitcham: Age Concern Research Unit.

Bhalla, A. and Blakemore, K. (1981) *Elders of Ethnic Minority Groups*, Birmingham: All Faiths For One Race.

Blakemore, K. (1983) 'Ethnicity, self-reported illness and use of medical services by the elderly', *Postgraduate Medical Journal* 59: 668–70.

Blaxter, M. (1976) *The Meaning of Disability*, London: Heinemann.

Bury, M.R. and Wood, P.H.N. (1978) 'Sociological perspectives in research on disablement', *International Rehabilitation Medicine* 1: 24–32.

Cook, J. and Watt, S. (1987) 'Racism, women and poverty', in C. Glendenning and J. Millar (eds) *Women and Poverty in Britain*, London: Tavistock.

Cornwell, J. (1984) *Hard Earned lives*, London: Tavistock.

Donaldson, L. (1986) 'Health and social status of elderly Asians: a community survey', *British Medical Journal* 293: 1079–82.

Donovan, J. (1986) *We Don't Buy Sickness, It Just Comes*, Aldershot: Gower Press.

Duckworth, D. (1983) *The Classification and Measurement of Disablement*, London: DHSS HMSO Research Report No. 10.

Ebrahim, S., Smith, C. and Giggs, J. (1987) 'Elderly immigrants — disadvantaged group?', *Age and Ageing* 16: 249–55.

Evers, H., Badger, F., Cameron, E., and Atkin, K. (forthcoming) *Community Care Project Working Papers*, Department of Social Medicine, University of Birmingham.

Fennell, G., Phillipson, C., and Evers, H. (1988) *The Sociology of Old Age*, Milton Keynes: Open University Press.

GLAD (1987) *Disability and Ethnic Minority Communities — a Study in Three London Boroughs*, London: Greater London Association for Disabled People.

Harris, A.I. with Cox, E. and Smith, C.R.W. (1971) *Handicapped and Impaired in Great Britain*, London: HMSO.

Holland, B. and Lewando-Hundt, G. (1987) *Coventry Ethnic Minorities Elderly Survey: Method, Data and Applied Action*, City of Coventry, Ethnic Minorities Development Unit.

247

Hunt, A. (1978) *The Elderly At Home*, London: HMSO.

Jefferys, M., Millard, J.B., Hyman, M., and Warren, M.D. (1969) 'A set of tests for measuring motor impairment in prevalence studies', *Journal for Chronic Diseases* 22: 303–19.

Johnson, M., Cross, M., and Cardew, S. (1983) 'Inner city residents, ethnic minorities and primary health care', *Postgraduate Medical Journal* 59: 664–7.

Locker, D. (1983) *Disability and Disadvantage: The Consequences of Chronic Illness*, London: Tavistock.

McFarland, E., Dalton, M., and Walsh, D. (1987) *Personal Welfare Services and Ethnic Minorities*, Research Paper No. 4, Scottish Ethnic Minority Research Unit, Glasgow College of Technology, Edinburgh College of Art and Herriot Watt University.

Norman, A. (1980) *Rights and Risk*, London: National Corporation for the Care of Old People.

Norman, A. (1985) *Triple Jeopardy: Growing Old in a Second Homeland*, London: Centre for Policy on Ageing.

Peace, S. (1986) 'The forgotten female: social policy and older women', in C. Phillipson and A. Walker (eds) *Ageing and Social Policy: A Critical Assessment*, Aldershot: Gower.

Phillipson, C. (1982) *Capitalism and the Construction of Old Age*, London: Macmillan.

RADAR (1984) *Disability and Minority Ethnic Groups: A Factsheet of Issues and Initiatives*, London: The Royal Association for Disability and Rehabilitation.

Townsend, P. (1967) *The Disabled in Society*, London: GLAD.

Townsend, P. (1981) 'The structured dependency of the elderly: a creation of social policy in the twentieth century', *Ageing and Society* 1: 5–28.

Townsend, P. and Davidson, N. (1982) *Inequalities in Health. The Black Report*, Harmondsworth: Penguin Books.

Walker, A. (1980) 'The social creation of poverty and dependency in old age', *Journal of Social Policy* 9: 172–88.

Whitehead, M. (1987) *The Health Divide: Inequalities in Health in the 1980s*, London: Health Education Authority.

Name Index

Subject Index

abuse: of alcohol 9, 16; of statistics 13, 17
activity rates: male/female 102-3
affluence 16-17, 115
Afro-Caribbean citizens 230, 231, 232, 236
After Redundancy study 73-88
Age Concern 225
Age Discrimination in Employment Act (1978) 65
age profile: Britain (1901-81) 1-3; socio-economic implications of 10-12
ageing/old people 7; as a burden 12, 21, 34, 36, 46, 51-2, 54, 225; in the church 158-9; demography of 1-10, 128; models of 157-8; population 1-18, 50, 128
ageism 84
alcohol abuse 9, 16
anthropological approaches to ageing 152, 171, 201
Asian citizens 230-47
asset ownership 68-9
Audit Commission report 186

Banfield John: House of Commons motion on pensions 31
behaviourist argument 9
Beveridge, William: Social Insurance Committee 30, 34-7, 38, 47, 117
Bevin, Ernest: retirement pension scheme, 31

black old women 230-48; and the NHS 244; isolation of 237; racism and 238
blaming the victim 12
brothers see siblings

care of old people/the elderly 46, 166-85, 186-200, 201-17, 218-29, 230-48 see also carers; community care; convalescence; discharge; general practitioners; home-help services; hospital discharge schemes; kin/kinship; meals-on-wheels; networks; paid helpers; residential homes; social services
carers 190-9, 230-48 see also care of old people/the elderly; community care; kinship; paid helpers
Central Birmingham Health Authority: research project 230, 233-4
Chamberlain, Neville: cost of retirement pensions 30
chiropody 96
clubs see old people's clubs
community care 222-3, 224, 227
Community Care Research Project 230, 232
convalescence 218-29
cross-cultural research problems 235-6

death, experiences of 211-12

253